IARC MONOGRAPHS

ON THE

EVALUATION OF THE CARCINOGENIC

RISK OF CHEMICALS TO MAN:

CERTAIN POLYCYCLIC AROMATIC HYDROCARBONS

AND

HETEROCYCLIC COMPOUNDS

Volume 3

This publication is the outcome of the
meeting of the IARC Working Group on
the Evaluation of the Carcinogenic Risk
of Chemicals to Man, Lyon, 5-11 December 1972

IARC WORKING GROUP ON THE EVALUATION OF THE CARCINOGENIC RISK OF CHEMICALS TO MAN: CERTAIN POLYCYCLIC AROMATIC HYDROCARBONS AND HETEROCYCLIC COMPOUNDS

Lyon, 5-11 December 1972

Members

Professor E. Boyland, 42, Bramerton Street, London SW3, UK

Professor W. Dontenwill, Forschungsinstitut der Zigaretten Industrie, Gazellenkamp 38, Hamburg, Federal Republic of Germany (Vice-Chairman)

Dr H.L. Falk, National Institutes of Environmental Health Sciences, Research Triangle Park, P.O. Box 12233, N.C. 27709, USA (Chairman)

Dr B.G. Gori, Associate Scientific Director for Program, Etiology, National Cancer Institute, National Institutes of Health, Bethesda, Maryland 20014, USA

Dr M.D. Kipling, Medical Adviser, Department of Employment, Somerset House, 37, Temple Street, Birmingham 2, UK

Dr R.W. Miller, Chief, Epidemiology Branch, A521 Landow Building, National Cancer Institute, National Institutes of Health, Bethesda, Maryland 20014, USA

Dr B. Terracini, Istituto di Anatomia e Istologie Patologica, Università di Torino, via Santena 7, 10126 Torino, Italy

Representative of the National Cancer Institute

Dr J. Cooper, Director, Information and Resources Segment, National Cancer Institute, National Institutes of Health, Bethesda, Maryland 20014, USA

Invited guests

Dr P.S. Elias, Principal Medical Officer, Department of Health and Social Security, Alexander Fleming House, Elephant and Castle, London SE1, UK

Dr H.P. Harke, Forschungsinstitut der Zigaretten Industrie, Gazellenkamp 38, Hamburg, Federal Republic of Germany

Secretariat

Dr C. Agthe, Unit of Chemical Carcinogenesis (Secretary)
Dr N. Breslow, Unit of Epidemiology and Biostatistics
Dr P. Bogovski, Unit of Environmental Carcinogens
Dr A.J. Cohen, IARC Consultant
Dr J. Higginson, Director
Dr R. Kratel, Occupational Health Unit, WHO
Mrs I. Peterschmitt, Unit of Chemical Carcinogenesis
Dr L. Tomatis, Unit of Chemical Carcinogenesis
Dr A.J. Tuyns, Unit of Epidemiology and Biostatistics
Mr E.A. Walker, Unit of Environmental Carcinogens

CONTENTS

	Page
BACKGROUND AND PURPOSE OF THE IARC PROGRAMME ON THE EVALUATION OF THE CARCINOGENIC RISK OF CHEMICALS TO MAN	7
SCOPE OF THE MONOGRAPHS	7
MECHANISM FOR PRODUCING THE MONOGRAPHS	8
Priority for the preparation of monographs	9
Data on which the evaluation was based	9
The Working Group	10
GENERAL REMARKS ON THE EVALUATION	10
Terminology	10
Response to carcinogens	10
Qualitative aspects	11
Quantitative aspects	11
Extrapolation from animals to man	12
Evidence of carcinogenicity to humans	12
Mixtures and groups of carcinogens	13
EXPLANATORY NOTES ON THE MONOGRAPHS	14
GENERAL REMARKS ON THE SUBSTANCES CONSIDERED	17
HISTORICAL REVIEW OF CANCER IN WORKERS EXPOSED TO POLYCYCLIC AROMATIC HYDROCARBONS AND HETEROCYCLIC COMPOUNDS AND THEIR ROLE IN OTHER ENVIRONMENTAL SITUATIONS	22
Soot and carbon black	22
Coal-tar and pitch	25

Contents (cont'd)

                                                                                          Page

    Mineral oils 30

    The role of polycyclic aromatic hydrocarbons and heterocyclic compounds in non-occupational exposure 34

THE MONOGRAPHS

    Polycyclic aromatic hydrocarbons:

        Benz(a)anthracene 45
        Benzo(b)fluoranthene 69
        Benzo(j)fluoranthene 82
        Benzo(a)pyrene 91
        Benzo(e)pyrene 137
        Chrysene 159
        Dibenz(a,h)anthracene 178
        Dibenzo(h,rst)pentaphene 197
        Dibenzo(a,e)pyrene 201
        Dibenzo(a,h)pyrene 207
        Dibenzo(a,i)pyrene 215
        Dibenzo(a,l)pyrene 224
        Indeno(1,2,3-cd)pyrene 229

    Heterocyclic compounds:

        Benz(c)acridine 241
        Dibenz(a,h)acridine 247
        Dibenz(a,j)acridine 254
        7H-dibenzo(c,g)carbazole 260

CUMULATIVE INDEX TO MONOGRAPHS 269

BACKGROUND AND PURPOSE OF THE IARC PROGRAMME ON THE EVALUATION OF THE CARCINOGENIC RISK OF CHEMICALS TO MAN

In the past few years the number and quantity of chemicals in the environment have increased. The possible adverse effect of these chemicals on human health is a matter of international concern. The International Agency for Research on Cancer (IARC) has consequently initiated a programme for the evaluation of the carcinogenic risk of chemicals to man, which was supported by a Resolution of the Governing Council at its Ninth Session concerning the role of the Agency in providing government authorities with expert, independent scientific opinion on environmental carcinogenesis. As one means to this end, the Governing Council recommended that the Agency should continue to prepare monographs on the carcinogenic risk of individual chemicals to man.

In view of the importance of this programme and in order to expedite the production of monographs, the National Cancer Institute of the United States has provided IARC with additional funds for this purpose.

The objective of this programme is to achieve and publish a balanced evaluation of data through the deliberations of an international group of experts in chemical carcinogenesis and to put into perspective the present state of knowledge with the final aim of evaluating the data in terms of possible human risk, as well as to indicate the need for research efforts to close the gaps in our knowledge.

SCOPE OF THE MONOGRAPHS

In 1972 the first volume of these monographs was published[1].

---

[1] International Agency for Research on Cancer (1972) *IARC on the Evaluation of Carcinogenic Risk of Chemicals to Man*, 1, Lyon

These monographs summarize the evidence for the carcinogenicity of individual chemicals in a condensed uniform manner for easy comparison. The data were compiled, reviewed and evaluated by a working group of experts. No recommendations are given concerning preventive measures or legislation, since these matters depend on risk-benefit evaluation which seems best made by individual governments and/or international agencies such as WHO and ILO.

The first volume covered a number of substances not belonging to a particular chemical group, and the second volume[1] contains monographs on some inorganic and organometallic compounds. The present volume is devoted to a number of polycyclic aromatic hydrocarbons and heterocyclic compounds.

As new data on chemicals for which monographs have already been written and new principles for evaluation become available, re-evaluation will be made at future meetings and revised monographs will be published as necessary. Special meetings can be called to evaluate important compounds for which the data are controversial and for which there seems to be an urgent need for action by public health authorities. The monographs will be distributed to international and governmental agencies, will be available to industries and scientists dealing with these chemicals, and will form the basis of advice from IARC on carcinogenesis from these substances.

MECHANISM FOR PRODUCING THE MONOGRAPHS

As a first step, a list of chemicals for possible consideration by the Working Group was established. IARC collected pertinent references regarding physico-chemical characteristics, use and occurrence, as well as biological data

---

[1] International Agency for Research on Cancer (1973) *IARC Monographs on the Evaluation of Carcinogenic Risk of Chemicals to Man*, 2, *Some Inorganic and Organometallic Compounds* (in press)

on these compounds. The material was summarized by an expert consultant or an IARC staff member, who prepared the first draft monograph, which in some cases was sent to another expert for comments. This draft was circulated to all members of the Working Group about two months before the meeting, at which further additions to and deletions from the data were agreed upon and a final version of comments and evaluation on each compound was adopted.

Priority for the Preparation of Monographs

Priority for consideration was given mainly to chemicals for which some adequate experimental evidence of carcinogenicity existed and/or for which there was evidence of human exposure. However, neither human exposure nor potential carcinogenicity could be judged until all the relevant data had been collected and examined in detail. The inclusion of a particular compound in a monograph did not necessarily mean that the substance was considered to be carcinogenic. Equally, the fact that a substance had not yet been considered did not imply that it was non-carcinogenic.

Data on which the Evaluation was Based

With regard to the biological data, only published articles or papers already accepted for publication were reviewed. Every effort was made to cover the whole literature, but some studies may have been overlooked inadvertently. Since the monographs contain only the relevant data the reader is unable to judge whether or not a particular work was considered. It is therefore important that research workers who are aware of important data which may change the evaluation make them available to the Unit of Chemical Carcinogenesis of the International Agency for Research on Cancer, Lyon, France, in order that they can be considered for a possible re-evaluation.

The Working Group

The members of the Working Group who participated in the consideration of particular substances are listed at the beginning of this publication. Each monograph bears a footnote indicating the date of the meeting at which it was considered. The members of the Working Group were invited by IARC to serve in their individual capacities as scientists, and not as representatives of their governments or of any institute to which they were affiliated.

GENERAL REMARKS ON THE EVALUATION

Terminology

The term "chemical carcinogenesis" in its widely accepted sense is used to indicate the induction or enhancement of neoplasia by chemicals. It is recognized that, in the strict etymological sense, this term means the induction of cancer. However, common usage has led to its employment to denote the induction of various types of neoplasm. The terms "tumourigen", "oncogen" and "blastomogen" have all been used synonymously with "carcinogen", although occasionally "tumourigen" has been used specifically to denote the induction of benign tumours.

Response to Carcinogens

For present practical purposes, in general, no distinction is made between the induction of tumours and the enhancement of tumour incidence, although it is noted that there may be fundamental differences in mechanisms that will eventually be elucidated.

The response to a carcinogen in experimental animals may be observed in several forms:

(a) as a significant increase in the frequency of one or several types of neoplasm, as compared to the control;

(b) as the occurrence of neoplasms not observed in control animals;
(c) as a decreased latent period as compared with control animals;
(d) as a combination of (a) and (c).

Qualitative Aspects

The qualitative nature of neoplasia has been much discussed. Many instances of carcinogenesis involve the induction of both benign and malignant tumours. There are few, if any, recorded instances in which only benign tumours are induced; their occurrence in experimental systems indicates that the same treatment may increase the risk of malignant tumours also.

In experimental carcinogenesis, the type of cancer seen is often the same as that recorded in human studies (e.g., bladder cancer in man, monkeys, dogs and hamsters after administration of 2-naphthylamine). In other instances, however, a chemical will induce different neoplasms or neoplasms at different sites in different animal species (e.g., benzidine, which induces hepatic carcinoma in the rat, but bladder carcinoma in man).

Purity of the compound tested

The Working Group was often faced with lack of information on the purity of the compounds tested. In order to render better judgement, whether the compound itself or the impurity is responsible for the carcinogenic effect, detailed specification of the substance under test is essential.

Quantitative Aspects

Dose-response studies are important in the evaluation of human and animal carcinogenesis. Sometimes, the only way in which a causal effect can be established with confidence is by the observation of increased incidence of neoplasms over the control in relation to increased exposure. It is hoped that, eventually, dose-response data may be used for assessment in carcinogenesis in the same way that they are used in general toxicological practice.

Extrapolation from Animals to Man

No attempt has been made to interpret the animal data in the absence of human data in terms of possible human risk, and no distinction has been made between weak and strong carcinogens, since no objective criteria are at present available to do so. These monographs may be reviewed if some such criteria should be elaborated. In the meantime, the critical assessment of the validity of the animal data given should help national and/or international authorities to make decisions concerning preventive measures or legislation in the light of WHO recommendations on food additives,[1] drugs[2] and occupational carcinogens[3].

Evidence of Carcinogenicity to Humans

Evidence that a particular chemical is carcinogenic in man depends on clinical and epidemiological data, which may be in the main descriptive, retrospective or prospective.

---

[1] World Health Organization (1961) Fifth Report of the Joint FAO/WHO Expert Committee on Food Additives. Evaluation of the carcinogenic hazards of food additives. Wld Hlth Org. techn. Rep. Ser., No. 220, pp. 5, 18 and 19

[2] World Health Organization (1964) Report of a WHO Expert Committee. Prevention of Cancer. Wld Hlth Org. techn. Rep. Ser., No. 276, pp. 29 and 30

[3] World Health Organization (1969) Report of a WHO Scientific Group. Principles for the testing and evaluation of drugs for carcinogenicity. Wld Hlth Org. techn. Rep. Ser., No. 426, pp. 19, 21 and 22

Descriptive studies may identify a cluster or a change in rates for a particular neoplasm in a subgroup of the population which suggests the influence of carcinogens in the environment. Retrospective studies (i.e., case-control studies that go into the histories of persons with or without cancer) have revealed occupational carcinogens (e.g., shale oil, chromates, asbestos, β-naphthylamine, benzidine) or iatrogenic carcinogens (e.g., chlornaphazin, thorotrast, diethylstilbestrol).

Once a relationship is known or suspected between an exposure and cancer, prospective studies (i.e., follow-up or cohort studies of exposed and unexposed groups) will identify more precisely the magnitude of the risk and may clarify time relationships, dose-response effects and other aspects of cancer induction. Whenever possible the Working Group considered evidence of the influence of variables other than the agent under suspicion in inducing the cancer under study (e.g., cigarette-smoking in the study of lung cancer among asbestos workers).

Finally, if man does develop cancer from a specific chemical, its removal from the environment should be followed eventually by epidemiological evidence of a decline in the frequency of the neoplasm in the exposed group.

Mixtures and Groups of Carcinogens

Mixtures of chemicals are sometimes associated with the occurrence of cancers in man, but no information is available on the specific components. Continuing efforts should be made to elucidate the role of the various components and impurities in substances to assist in planning better preventive measures and to provide a basis for assessing similar hazards. There are situations where carcinogens may occur in groups in the human environment and where it is not yet possible to attribute the observed effects to individual substances. This is notably so in the case of the polycyclic aromatic hydrocarbons, heterocyclic compounds and certain aromatic amines.

EXPLANATORY NOTES ON THE MONOGRAPHS

In sections 1, 2 and 3 of each monograph, except for minor remarks, the data are recorded as given by the author, whereas the comments by the Working Group are given in section 4, headed "Comments on data reported and evaluation".

Title of the Monograph

The monograph has as its title the chemical name of the substance under consideration. For this name, the chemical abstract nomenclature is normally used.

Chemical and Physical Data (section 1)

Chemical and physical properties include data that might be relevant to carcinogenicity (for example, lipid solubility) and those that concern identification. Where relevant, data on solubility, volatility and stability are indicated. All data except those for "Technical products and impurities" refer to the pure substances.

Use and Occurrence (section 2)

The analytical data recorded under "Occurrence" are dependent on the methods employed. In some instances the quantitative and even the qualitative results may be questionable because the methods were not satisfactory. Data on human exposure are also included, where available, under this heading.

Biological Data Relevant to the Evaluation of Carcinogenic Risk to Man (section 3)

As pointed out earlier in this introduction, the monographs are not intended to itemize all studies reported in the literature. Although every effort was made to review the whole literature, some studies were purposely omitted (a) because of their inadequacy[1,2,3] (e.g., too short a duration, too few animals, poor survival or too small a dose), (b) because they only confirmed findings already reported or (c) because they were judged irrelevant for the purpose of the evaluation. The data recorded here are summarized as given by the author; however, certain shortcomings of reporting or of experimental design are also mentioned, and minor comments by the Working Group are given in brackets. The essential critical comments by the Working Group are, however, made in section 4 ("Comments on data reported and evaluation").

Carcinogenicity and related studies in animals (3.1)

Mention is made of all routes of administration by which the compound has been tested and all species in which the chemical has been investigated. In some cases where similar results were obtained by other authors and/or other laboratories, reference is made to a summary article. Quantitative

---

[1] World Health Organization (1958) Second Report of the Joint FAO/WHO Expert Committee on Food Additives. Procedures for the testing of intentional food additives to establish their safety for use. Wld Hlth Org. techn. Rep. Ser., No. 144

[2] World Health Organization (1961) Fifth Report of the Joint FAO/WHO Expert Committee on Food Additives. Evaluation of the carcinogenic hazards of food additives. Wld Hlth Org. techn. Rep. Ser., No. 220

[3] World Health Organization (1967) Scientific Group. Procedures for investigating intentional and unintentional food additives. Wld Hlth Org. techn. Rep. Ser., No. 348

data are given in so far as they will enable the reader to realize the order of magnitude of the effective dose. In some cases, where in the same experiments other polycyclic aromatic hydrocarbons were investigated, parallel results on these were also included to compare their biological activity with the substance in question. The doses are indicated as they appear in the original paper. In general, negative experiments of an inadequate standard[1] are not summarized. In certain cases, however, it was felt that such data should be included since they would contribute to the total picture.

Other relevant biological data (3.2)

The data reported in this section are divided into three categories: (a) information on the metabolic fate in animals including localization into tissues, (b) similar information on man and (c) comparison of animal and human data. Data on acute toxicity are included when considered relevant.

Observations in man (3.3)

Epidemiological studies are summarized. This subsection also includes, where relevant, summaries of reports of cases of cancer in man that have been related to possible exposure to the chemical.

Comments on Data Reported and Evaluation (section 4)

This section includes the critical view of the Working Group on the data reported. It is purposely kept as brief as possible since it should be read in conjunction with the data recorded.

---

[1] World Health Organization (1961) Fifth Report of the Joint FAO/WHO Expert Committee on Food Additives. Evaluation of the carcinogenic hazards of food additives. Wld Hlth Org. techn. Rep. Ser., No. 220

Animal data (4.1)

The animal species mentioned are those in which the carcinogenicity of the substances was clearly demonstrated, irrespective of the route of administration. In the case of inadequate studies, when mentioned, comments to that effect are included. The route of administration used in experimental animals that is similar to the possible human exposure (ingestion, inhalation and skin exposure) is given particular mention. In most cases, tumour sites are also indicated. Comparison of the carcinogenic activity with that of other polycyclic aromatic hydrocarbons was made in some cases in which parallel experiments were run in the same study. If the substance has produced tumours on pre-natal exposure or in single-dose experiments, this is also indicated. This subsection should be read in the light of comments made in the section "Extrapolation from animals to man" of this introduction.

Human data (4.2)

In some cases, a brief statement is made on the possible exposure of man. The significance of epidemiological studies and case reports is discussed, and the data are interpreted in terms of possible human risk.

GENERAL REMARKS ON THE SUBSTANCES CONSIDERED

This volume of monographs is devoted to a number of polycyclic aromatic hydrocarbons (PAH) and heterocyclic compounds which were selected on the basis of experimental evidence of their carcinogenicity in animals by an earlier IARC Working Group.

Important biological considerations

Because epidemiological studies have been conducted in environmental situations where these compounds are encountered as mixtures, often ill-defined, rather than as pure substances, the 1971 Working Group recommended that the epidemiological data should be presented as an individual section in a volume devoted to polycyclic aromatic hydrocarbons and heterocyclic compounds. For this reason, a preamble to these monographs was incorporated by the present Working Group. It is not the intention of these monographs to direct attention to any particular aromatic hydrocarbon or group of aromatic hydrocarbons as specifically related to human cancer, but simply to assess them individually on the available data. Other factors not fully understood may contribute to this relationship, among them synergistic and anticarcinogenic effects.

<u>Environmental data</u>

In many laboratories environmental analyses include both carcinogenic and non-carcinogenic polycyclic aromatic hydrocarbons and heterocyclic compounds. A joint UICC/IARC meeting in 1968[1] decided that an acceptable method should be capable of separating and estimating at least benzo(a)pyrene, dibenz(a,h)anthracene, dibenz(a,h)acridine, benzo(g,h,i)perylene, pyrene and coronene; the latter three compounds were considered non-carcinogenic by the above-mentioned committee and are not included in this volume.

The Working Group at the IARC meeting concerned with the standardization of procedures for the estimation of polycyclic aromatic hydrocarbons in air[2] decided that the following compounds should be looked for: benzo(a)pyrene, benzo(e)pyrene, benzo(k)fluoranthene, benzo(g,h,i)perylene, coronene and

---

[1] UICC (1970) <u>The quantification of environmental carcinogens</u> (UICC Technical Report Series, Vol. 4)

[2] International Agency for Research on Cancer (1971) <u>Standardization of sampling and analytical procedures for estimation of polynuclear hydrocarbons in the environment.</u> IARC internal techn. Rep., No. 71/002

benz(a)anthracene. The Working Group included benzo(k)fluoranthene and benzo(g,h,i)perylene because in some analytical procedures they interfered with the determination of benzo(a)pyrene and had to be quantitated at the same time as the carcinogen. Benz(a)anthracene was included because of its carcinogenicity, although quantitative determination would be difficult because of its volatility. Analysis for pyrene was not accepted for reasons of volatility.

Table I illustrates the variation in selection of compounds to be analyzed by different groups and laboratories studying a range of environmental aspects.

TABLE I

	UICC (1970)	IARC (1971)	WHO (1970)	Stocks et al. (1961)	Waller & Commins (1967)	Borneff & Kunte (1969)	Grimmer & Hildebrandt (1965)	Howard et al. (1966)
Benzo(a)pyrene	D	D	D	D	D	D	D	D
Benzo(e)pyrene	-	D	-	D	D	-	D	D
Benzo(k)fluoranthene	-	D	D	-	-	D	D	-
Benzo(g,h,i)perylene	D	D	D	D	D	D	D	D
Coronene	D	D	-	D	D	-	D	-
Benz(a)anthracene	-	D	-	-	-	D	D	D
Dibenz(a,h)anthracene	D	-	-	-	-	-	D	-
Dibenz(a,h)acridine	D	-	-	-	-	-	-	-
Pyrene	D	-	-	D	-	-	D	-
Anthanthrene	-	-	-	D	-	-	D	-
Fluoranthene	-	-	D	D	-	D	D	-
Perylene	-	-	-	-	-	-	D	-
Benzo(b)fluoranthene	-	-	D	-	-	D	-	-
Indeno(1,2,3-cd)pyrene	-	-	D	-	-	D	-	-
Phenanthrene	-	-	-	-	-	-	D	-
Chrysene	-	-	-	-	-	-	D	-
Anthracene	-	-	-	-	-	-	D	-

D - Selected for quantitative determination

Analytical methods applicable to a number of polycyclic hydrocarbons

Adequate and reliable methods for the detection and quantitative determination of polycyclic aromatic hydrocarbons in environmental and in biological samples are available.

Generally, environmental trace analysis procedures may be subdivided into (a) sampling, (b) separation from the substrate, (c) "clean-up" and concentration and (d) determination. These subdivisions are of course not rigid; e.g., gas chromatography can achieve isolation and quantitation simultaneously.

For the compounds considered, procedures in (a) may range from the comparatively standardized sampling of food to the complex problem of collecting fine airborne particulate matter. Procedures in (b) may include sublimation, distillation, solid-liquid or liquid-liquid extraction. Those in (c) involve one or more chromatographic techniques, including liquid-column, thin-layer and paper chromatography, application of which has been extensively reviewed (Sawicki, 1964; Schaad, 1970). In (d), ultra-violet absorption and fluorescence spectrophotometry are commonly employed, but gas chromatography and its combination with mass spectrometry are finding increasing application particularly where detailed analysis is required (Sawicki, 1964; Schaad, 1970). The rapidly developing technique of high-pressure liquid chromatography is also being explored (Jentoft & Gouw, 1968) and may find useful application for the separation and analysis of PAH.

The UICC Report (1970) examines the general policy of PAH analysis. A general method for the analysis of total diet composites has been developed by Howard et al. (1968), and reviews of PAH analysis include that of van Langermeersch (1968).

Comprehensive instructions for the determination of PAH in air have been elaborated by Sawicki et al. (1970).

The Working Group felt reluctant to indicate limits of detection for the various methods used in the quantitative determination of polycyclic aromatic hydrocarbons because the sensitivity of a particular method may vary according to the sample to be analyzed and the preliminary steps taken in the preparation of the samples.

Solubility

The polycyclic aromatic hydrocarbons exhibit a wide range of solubilities in organic solvents. They are generally more soluble in nitromethane and in aromatic solvents such as benzene and toluene than in the lower aliphatic alcohols such as ethanol. Their solubility in aliphatic hydrocarbon solvents usually falls between the two groups above. The heterocyclic compounds considered tend to be more soluble in alcohol than do the PAH. All are insoluble or very sparingly soluble in water. Solubility characteristics are usefully employed in separation and analysis.

Estimates of atmospheric exposure

The Working Group was confronted with a large amount of widely varying data on the quantities of polycyclic aromatic hydrocarbons present in air from many localities under various conditions, such as season, traffic density, general pollution level, etc. and using various methodology and sampling techniques. The data are condensed to give the reader useful information, but no estimates of the daily atmospheric intake of PAH and heterocyclic compounds by the general population were made.

HISTORICAL REVIEW OF CANCER IN WORKERS EXPOSED TO POLYCYCLIC AROMATIC HYDROCARBONS AND HETEROCYCLIC COMPOUNDS AND THEIR ROLE IN OTHER ENVIRONMENTAL SITUATIONS

Because polycyclic aromatic hydrocarbons are so well established experimentally as carcinogens, it is important to evaluate their capacity to induce cancer in man. There is a wealth of information concerning the effects of these chemicals on various tissues and organs of laboratory animals. In man, however, exposures have not been to individual chemicals but to combinations as they occur in soot, coal-tar, pitch and mineral oils, and also in environmental substances including tobacco smoke and exhaust. Environmental exposures to these substances are thus considered here separately from the monographs concerning the carcinogenicity of individual aromatic polycyclic hydrocarbons.

In this section human data, animal experiment data and chemical composition are examined in that order, since this is how our knowledge developed historically.

1. SOOT AND CARBON BLACK

1.1 Human data

Soot was first noted as a cause of skin cancer in man when Pott (1775) wrote that the disease "seems to derive its origin from a lodgment of soot in the rugae of the scrotum". Subsequently, cancer in chimney sweeps was described elsewhere on the skin and in internal organs (Butlin, 1892a).

It has been observed more recently (Sulman & Sulman, 1946) that soot formed by burning wood produced very little benzo(a)-pyrene when compared with coal soot. The evidence for a relationship between exposure to soot and skin cancer was supported by the reduction of incidence of scrotal cancer in chimney sweeps after the institution of control measures in

Great Britain (Schamberg, 1910). Skin cancer appeared in workers between eight and 47 years of age; whereas cancers following exposure to paraffin or tar occurred mainly in those between 34 and 60 years of age (Liebe, 1892). The 22-year difference in age at onset can be accounted for in part by the early age at which the chimney sweep began his apprenticeship: it was not uncommon for such service to begin at four years of age (Butlin, 1892b).

Commercially prepared soot, known as carbon black, produced no increase in cancer risk among workers (Ingalls, 1950; Tara, 1960); but cases have been described in the mixing of carbon black and oil in the rubber industry (Henry, 1946).

The apparent discrepancies in old and recent literature concerning the incidence of cancer following occupational contact with soot or carbon black are generally explained by new technology, advances in hygiene and enforcement of industrial legislation.

1.2 Animal data

The experimental production of skin cancer with extracts of soot was accomplished first by Passey (1922), who found that the most potent extracts were those which were free of acidic and phenolic compounds. He suggested that earlier unsuccessful attempts at tumour induction were due to lack of contact, penetration or duration of exposure to soot, to inappropriate samples of soot, or to inappropriate choice of the animal species tested.

The reported inability to induce cancer in mice by feeding carbon black (Nau et al., 1958a) or by applying it to the skin (Nau et al., 1958b) was overcome by administering solvent extracts by injection or by skin-painting (Falk & Steiner, 1952; Von Haam & Mallette, 1952). A benzene extract of oil shale soot (0.01% benzo(a)pyrene) mixed with Tween 60 produced lung cancer after intratracheal instillation in rats (Bogovski et al., 1970).

PAH have been identified in carbon black, processed rubber and rubber tyre extracts which were carcinogenic for mice (Fålk et al., 1951).

1.3 Chemical composition

Benzo(a)pyrene is quantitatively the most important compound present in soot, although some other carcinogenic PAH have been detected in small amounts. It is not only a potent carcinogen, but also one for which the largest number of analytical methods is available.

Industrially, the synthesis of PAH is largely dependent upon specific procedures in which the combustion temperature of the organic matter determines the reaction products. In the range of 1100-1600°C organic compounds break down and, in the absence of sufficient oxygen, cracking occurs, with the release of hydrogen, carbon and CH radicals (Ellis, 1937). Polymerization of these free radicals takes place via "nascent acetylene", a term coined by Groll (1933).

Soot can contain benzo(a)pyrene, other carcinogenic compounds and compounds that are not carcinogenic. The carcinogens other than benzo(a)pyrene are of considerable interest with respect to their effect in man. They may contribute to the apparent contradictions in the literature concerning the variable cancer-producing activity of soot.

Falk & Steiner (1952) showed that carbon blacks of the furnace-black type contain several polycyclic aromatic hydrocarbons; the following seven were identified: pyrene, fluoranthene, benzo(a)pyrene, benzo(e)pyrene, anthanthrene, benzo(g,h,i)perylene and coronene, and are readily extractable by a number of solvents from soot having an average particle diameter of 40 mµ or more (Kotin & Falk, 1959). The same compounds were extractable only in trace amounts from smaller sized particles; whereas none were obtained from channel blacks, which are prepared by a different process which yields particles of between 10 and 30 mµ average diameter. These substances do not release polycyclic hydrocarbons on solvent extraction but will absorb them from solution (Falk & Steiner, 1952).

Improvements in analytical techniques have increased the number of PAH detectable in carbon black. The newly identified compounds (including several benzofluoranthenes) do not appear to contribute significantly to the carcinogenic activity since they are either non-carcinogenic or, if carcinogenic, are present in small quantities. The inability to estimate the carcinogenic properties of "soot" or to evaluate the exposure risk associated with its industrial use can be appreciated when one contrasts a channel black from which no benzo(a)pyrene can be eluted with incinerator soot from which 2 mg benzo(a)-pyrene/g of soot, i.e., 0.2%, were obtained (Sawicki, 1962).

2. COAL-TAR AND PITCH

2.1 Human data

Butlin (1892c) described skin cancer among workers in the coal-tar and pitch industry. Largely through publications by Henry (1946, 1947) it was realized that the differing composition of tar products was related to the frequency of skin cancer among coal-tar workers. In 1907, the Workman's Compensation Act in England recognized officially that cutaneous epitheliomas could be caused by pitch or tarry substances. Ross (1948) classified the products obtained on distillation of coal-tar as shown in Table II:

TABLE II

Temperature	Compounds Produced
– 170°C	light oils; benzene, toluene, xylene
170° – 230°C	middle oils; phenols, cresols, naphthalene
230° – 270°C	creosote oils, tar oils
270° – 400°C	anthracene oils
	pitch residue

Exposures to pitch occur not only among coal-tar workers, but also among optical lens grinders, electrical equipment workers and wharfmen, cable layers, net fixers and fabric proofers (Jenkins, 1948). Exposure to creosote oil occurs among brick and tile workers, as well as among timber-proofers (Henry, 1946).

In contrast with cancer occurring in chimney sweeps, occupational exposure to tar and pitch affects predominantly skin sites other than the scrotum. From 1920-45, pitch or tar was deemed responsible for 2229 of 3753 notified industrial skin cancers in Great Britain (Henry, 1946, 1947); while during the decade 1946-55, 2041 new cases of occupational skin cancer were notified in Great Britain, of which 1053 were attributed to tar and pitch (Bogovski, 1960).

The majority of skin cancers in tar workers have been reported from England, but other reports have come from USA (Heller, 1930), Holland (de Vries, 1928), Germany (Volkmann, 1875) and France (Manouvriez, 1876).

Human skin cancers have been described after exposures to creosote oil (O'Donovan, 1928; Cookson, 1924; Lenson, 1956) and to anthracene oil (Bridge & Henry, 1928; O'Donovan, 1921).

Kennaway & Kennaway (1947) described an increased frequency of lung cancer among workers exposed to coal gas and tar. Doll (1952) found that among 2071 male pensioners of a London gas company, the number of deaths from lung cancers was approximately double that expected for male inhabitants of London of the same age (25 deaths observed vs 13.8 expected). The investigation concerned a multiplicity of occupations within the company, and it is probable that the risk was substantially greater for men most closely concerned with gas production.

In a further study, Doll et al. (1972) examined the mortality experience of groups of gas-workers in Great Britain over a period of 12 years. Among those categorized as coal carbonizing process workers, they found a significant excess of deaths from lung cancer (3.82 vs 2.13 per 100 000 per year); the rates for bladder cancer (0.40 vs 0.17) and cancer of skin and scrotum (0.12 vs 0.02) were also significantly higher than the national rates. Work as topman appeared to be particularly hazardous. The risk for lung cancer could not be related to any particular type of retort house. Among the by-products workers, there was no substantial evidence of any specific occupational hazard.

In Japan, 21 men exposed to coal-tar fumes in generator-gas plants developed lung cancer in a six-year period, a seeming excess over normal expectation (Kuroda & Kawahata, 1936). Kawai et al. (1967) observed that the longer the exposure the greater was the mortality from lung cancer, beginning ten years after exposure to coal-tar fumes.

In a British study of retort houses, certain areas were found to have 3 µg/m^3 benzo(a)pyrene, which was very much higher than the mean annual level for the city of London, away from the traffic, up to 1965. In the air above the retorts in the old horizontal retort houses where the processing temperature was 800 to 1000°C, the concentration of benzo(a)-pyrene was over 200 µg/m³. Such high levels were not found in vertical retort houses where the processing temperature was only 400 to 500°C (Lawther et al., 1965).

In a study of 58 528 employees of an American steelworks, Lloyd (1971) found that the mortality from respiratory cancer among coke plant workers was double that for steel workers as a whole. The excess was greater among those who had been employed directly at the ovens, particularly at the top of the ovens, among whom 15 lung cancer deaths occurred versus 1.5 expected.

Emissions from coke-ovens in the United States were analyzed for polycyclic aromatic hydrocarbons in 20 coke plants, and although their levels varied in each plant, similar ratios between benzo(a)pyrene, chrysene and benz(a)anthracene were found (Smith, 1970). In a report on a legal action involving one worker who developed lung cancer after working with tar, it was estimated that he could have inhaled 320 µg benzo(a)-pyrene per hour. The tar contained 3% benzo(a)pyrene and gave off vapours at 300°C containing 4.4% benzo(a)pyrene (Bonnet, 1962).

2.2 Animal data

Crude coal-tar was first shown to be carcinogenic experimentally by Yamagiwa & Ichikawa (1915) who painted it on rabbits' ears for several months; and later Tsutsui (1918) and Murray (1921) produced similar results on the skin of mice. Coal-tar pitch and anthracene oil, fractions of coal-tar, were also shown to be carcinogenic (Kennaway, 1925); Bonser (1932) produced skin cancers by administration of blast furnace tar. Twort & Fulton (1930) demonstrated that the carcinogenic potency of tars prepared at temperatures of 500°C, 600°C and 750°C increased materially with the temperature of preparation.

Lijinsky et al. (1957) have found commercial creosote oils to be highly carcinogenic. They contained 2.75 g/l benz(a)-anthracene, which is carcinogenic in the mouse (see monograph), and 1.27 g/l chrysene, a carcinogen for the mouse skin (see monograph). Benzo(a)pyrene and other pentacyclic PAH were present at much lower concentrations, i.e., about 50 mg/l.

2.3 Chemical composition

In an attempt to identify the responsible agent, carcinogenic coal-tar was fractionated and the aromatic fraction was found to be active. It possessed fluorescence, which led to the isolation and identification of benz(a)anthracene, a PAH with a characteristic fluorescence spectrum. On the basis of these findings, Kennaway & Hieger (1930), utilizing fluorescence spectroscopy, succeeded in isolating benzo(a)pyrene, which later proved to be carcinogenic, from coal-tar. With improved techniques, other PAH were isolated, among which dibenzo(a,h)-pyrene, dibenzo(a,i)pyrene, benzo(b)fluoranthene and dibenz(a,h)-anthracene (Badger, 1962) were also shown to be carcinogenic constitutents.

Kennaway (1925) manufactured carcinogenic tars synthetically from a variety of sources such as isoprene, acetylene, skin, yeasts and cholesterol, and showed that carcinogenicity increased with the temperature involved in the distillation of tars.

Tar produced by pyrolysis of acetylene contained 2% benzo(a)pyrene (Badger et al., 1960), and evidence has been presented for the pyrolytic formation of all known PAH encountered in soot (Badger, 1962). At 600-800°C, a yield of 0.1% to 0.15% of benzo(a)pyrene has been obtained through pyrolysis from isoprene (Gil-Av & Shabtai, 1963); the carcinogenic compound, dibenzo(a,i)pyrene, can be made from

3-vinyl-cyclohexene at 700°C (Badger & Novotny, 1961). Oil shale tar produced at 400-500°C contains 0.001-0.02% benzo(a)-pyrene (Bogovski, 1961).

3. MINERAL OILS

3.1 Human data

Volkmann (1875) described scrotal cancers among workers producing paraffin by the distillation of coal-tar. Subsequently, Liebe (1892) noted the absence of such hazard among workers exposed to pure paraffin. Several investigators have since shown that cancers among paraffin workers are not due to the paraffin but to impurities in oils produced during processing (Leitch, 1922; Hendricks et al., 1959). Refined paraffin is free of PAH and does not induce skin cancer in mice (Shubik et al., 1962).

Bell (1876) first described cancer of the scrotum in a Scottish shale oil worker. In a 23-year period, 49 Scottish paraffin workers developed skin cancer of which 13 were scrotal (Henry, 1946).

The cotton mule spinning industry in Great Britain originally used shale oil for the lubrication of the spindles (Henry, 1946). The first case of death from scrotal cancer in a worker who used shale oil in mule spinning occurred in 1923 (Bridge & Henry, 1928). In the years 1920 to 1943, there were 1303 legally notified cases of skin cancer in the British mule spinning industry, including 824 of the scrotum. There were 575 fatal cases of scrotal cancer recorded between 1911 and 1938 (Henry, 1946).

In Great Britain, the Mule Spinning Regulations have ensured that since 1953 only oil drastically refined with sulphuric acid shall be used in mule spinning and that mule spinners shall be medically examined every six months. These measures, together with the marked decline of the process of mule spinning, have produced a sustained fall in the incidence of cancer of the scrotum in Great Britain.

Cutting oils used by workers to cut metals were found to increase the risk of skin cancer in Birmingham, England (Cruickshank & Squire, 1950; Cruickshank & Gourevitch, 1952), particularly among workers in automatic machine shops. Between 1950 and 1967, 187 cases of scrotal cancer occurred in this region, of which at least two-thirds could be attributed to oil (Waterhouse, 1971).

At the present time toolsetters and setter operators in automatic shops who use heat cutting oil have an increased risk of cancer. The work requires constant contact with the machines and consequent contamination with the oil. In the Birmingham area of England, a high frequency of skin and scrotal cancer from oil has occurred, particularly among bar automatic machine workers; but other engineering practices also present a cancer hazard, e.g., metal rolling, tube drawing, metal hardening and machine operating. Although the major risk is from exposure to undiluted oils, emulsions have been incriminated occasionally. The industries most affected are those with automatic shops, such as nut and bolt manufacturers. Workers have also been affected after exposure during the changing of transformer oil in electrical sub-stations and during the painting or spraying of mould oil for brick- and tile-making or concrete moulding, in drop forging, rubber mixing, wire drawing, rope making and in the jute industry and from grease in metal working (Kipling, 1968).

In France, in the valley of the river Arve in the Savoy Alps, there have occurred since 1955 at least 60 cases of cancer of the scrotum together with many cases of cancer of the skin among the bar automatic machine workers (décolleteurs). The very high frequency in the relatively small population of the valley was observed mainly among the self-employed and workers in small premises (Thony & Thony, 1970). They were in contact with undiluted cutting oils.

Cancers of the larynx, lung and stomach have also been attributed to oil mist (Southam, 1928); and recently evidence has been produced that persons who developed cancer of the scrotum are significantly more liable to develop cancers at other sites, e.g., in the respiratory tract or upper digestive tract (Holmes et al., 1970).

3.2 Animal data

Leitch (1922) applied crude shale oil to mice and obtained tumour formation in the skin of 30 of the 74 mice that survived over 100 days. "Petroleum" oils were found to be less carcinogenic (Twort & Twort, 1931). Bingham & Horton (1966) showed that distillates of cutting oil are carcinogenic for the skin of mice even after sulphuric acid extraction; however, when they are extracted with furfural they become non-carcinogenic for mice over 80 weeks of skin application.

3.3 Chemical data

Mineral oils vary in their carcinogenicity and in their composition. Of particular interest are carcinogenic mineral oils that lack benzo(a)pyrene. Cook et al. (1958) isolated and identified components of various mineral oils, taking great care not to produce additional carcinogens during heating. In distilling below 250°C under reduced pressure, they produced a fraction free of benzo(a)pyrene which was carcinogenic for mice and rabbits in skin painting experiments. This observation was confirmed by Bogovski (1959) in benzo(a)pyrene-free fractions of shale oil. The individual compounds which were separated included di- tri-, and tetramethylphenanthrenes, tetramethylfluorene, methylpyrene, benzo(a)fluorene and several heterocyclic compounds, such as dimethyldibenzothiophene, dimethylnaphthothiophene and pentamethylcarbazole.

The carcinogenicity of mineral oil increases as the temperature is increased, as cracking occurs to form other compounds. Hueper & Cahnmann (1958) compared fractions with low and high boiling points, excluding those with benzo(a)pyrene, and found activity in six of them. One may conclude that mineral oils have various carcinogenic potencies depending on their origin, composition and treatment, and that some of the carcinogens may be three- or four-ring polycyclic aromatic hydrocarbons. Some of the fractions with carcinogenic activity may contain aliphatic hydrocarbons like dodecane, which possesses cocarcinogenic properties (Smith et al., 1951).

Other work (Badger, 1962) revealed that benzofluoranthenes, some of which are carcinogenic, are also present.

A report of the Medical Research Council (1968) stated that the carcinogenicity of crude oils appears to lie in impurities which boil above 350°C. From this fraction over 40 chemical compounds were isolated, several structurally similar to potent carcinogens. Compounds isolated included a wide range of aromatic hydrocarbons, e.g., di-, tri- and tetramethylnaphthalenes and phenanthrenes, chrysene and methyl derivatives, perylene, triphenylene and tetramethylfluorene. Heterocyclic compounds included di- and tetramethyldibenzothiophenes, thiobenzofluorene and tetra- and pentamethylcarbazoles.

The carcinogenicity of methyl derivatives of polycyclic and heterocyclic aromatic compounds will be considered in subsequent monographs.

4. THE ROLE OF PAH AND HETEROCYCLIC COMPOUNDS IN NON-OCCUPATIONAL EXPOSURE

PAH occur in many environmental situations (e.g., air, tobacco smoke or food) as a result of incomplete combustion, but their carcinogenic hazard to man cannot be estimated at present. The environmental exposure levels indicate that the hazard is relatively small compared with those found in certain occupations. However, this does not take into account the synergistic effects of other substances which might be present.

Satisfactory human epidemiological evidence is available concerning the synergistic effects of asbestos exposure and cigarette smoking, as well as for exposures to uranium ore dust and smoking.

Experimental confirmation of such synergistic effect is provided by the results of skin painting in mice, in which a 100-fold increase in skin cancer production has been observed when cigarette smoke condensate and equivalent benzo(a)pyrene concentrations were compared (Wynder & Hoffmann, 1967). As another example, a synergistic effect of dodecane and related substances on skin tumour induction in mice has been clearly demonstrated to be about 1000-fold for benzo(a)pyrene and about 100-fold for benz(a)anthracene (see monographs).

It is, therefore, obvious that no prediction as to human cancer risks can be made from a simple knowledge of the levels of PAH existing in the environment.

References

Badger, G.M. (1962) Mode of formation of carcinogens in human environment. Nat. Cancer Inst. Monogr., 9, 1

Badger, G.M. & Novotny, J. (1961) The formation of aromatic hydrocarbons at high temperatures: XIII. The pyrolysis of 3-vinylcyclohexene. J. chem. Soc., 3403

Badger, G.M., Lewis, G.E. & Napier, I.M. (1960) The formation of aromatic hydrocarbons at high temperatures: VIII. The pyrolysis of acetylene. J. chem. Soc., 2825

Bell, J. (1876) Paraffin epithelioma of the scrotum. Edin. med. J., 22, 135

Bingham, E. & Horton, A.W. (1966) Environmental carcinogenesis: Experimental observations related to occupational cancer. Advanc. Biol. Skin, 7, 183

Bogovski, P. (1959) Occupational skin tumours induced by products of thermal treatment of mineral fuels. Vop. Onkol., 5, 486

Bogovski, P. (1960) Occupational skin tumours due to fuel processing products. Leningrad, Medgiz

Bogovski, P. (1961) The cancerogenic effect of Estonian oil-shale processing products. Tallinn, Estonian Academy of Sciences

Bogovski, P., Vosamae, A. & Mirme, H. (1970) Cocarcinogenicity studies on oil-shale processing products. In: Tenth International Cancer Congress, Houston, Abstracts, p. 76

Bonnet, J. (1962) Quantitative analysis of benzo(a)pyrene in vapours coming from melted tar. Nat. Cancer Inst. Monogr., 9, 221

Bonser, G.M. (1932) Tumours of the skin produced by blast-furnace tar. Lancet, i, 775

Borneff, J. & Kunte, H. (1969) Kanzerogene Substanzen in Wasser und Boden. XXVI. Routinemethode zur Bestimmung von polyzyklischen Aromaten in Wasser. Arch. Hyg. (Muenchen), 147, 401

Bridge, J.C. & Henry, S.A. (1928) Industrial cancers. In: Report of the International Conference on Cancer, London, Bristol, John Wright, p. 258

Butlin, H.T. (1892a) Three lectures on cancer of the scrotum in chimney sweeps and others. I. Secondary cancer without primary cancer. Brit. med. J., i, 1341

Butlin, H.T. (1892b) Three lectures on cancer of the scrotum in chimney sweeps and others. II. Why foreign sweeps do not suffer from scrotal cancer. Brit. med. J., ii, 1

Butlin, H.T. (1892c) Three lectures on cancer of the scrotum in chimney sweeps and others. III. Tar and paraffin cancer. Brit. med. J., ii, 66

Cook, J.W., Carruthers, W. & Woodhouse, D.L. (1958) Carcinogenicity of mineral oil fractions. Brit. med. Bull., 14, 132

Cookson, H.A. (1924) Epithelioma of the skin after prolonged exposure to creosote. Brit. med. J., i, 368

Cruickshank, C.N.D. & Gourevitch, A. (1952) Skin cancer of the hand and forearm. Brit. J. industr. Med., 9, 74

Cruickshank, C.N.D. & Squire, J.R. (1950) Skin cancer in the engineering industry from the use of mineral oil. Brit. J. industr. Med., 7, 1

Doll, R. (1952) The causes of death among gas-workers with special reference to cancer of the lung. Brit. J. industr. Med., 9, 180

Doll, R., Vessey, M.P., Beasley, R.W.R., Buckley, A.R., Fear, E.C., Fisher, R.E.W., Gammon, E.J., Gunn, W., Hughes, G.O., Lee, K. & Norman-Smith, B. (1972) Mortality of gas-workers - final report of a prospective study. Brit. J. industr. Med., 29, 394

Ellis, C. (1937) The chemistry of petroleum derivatives, Vol. 2, New York, Reinhold

Falk, H.L. & Steiner, P.E. (1952) The identification of aromatic polycyclic hydrocarbons in carbon blacks. Cancer Res., 12, 30

Falk, H.L., Steiner, P.E., Goldfein, S., Breslow, A. & Hykes, R. (1951) Carcinogenic hydrocarbons and related compounds in processed rubber. Cancer Res., 11, 318

Gil-Av, E. & Shabtai, J. (1963) Precursors of carcinogenic hydrocarbons in tobacco smoke. Nature (Lond.), 197, 1065

Grimmer, G. & Hildebrandt, A. (1965) Kohlenwasserstoffe in der Umgebung der Menschen. I. Eine Methode zur simultanen Bestimmung von dreizehn polycyclischen Kohlenwasserstoffen. J. Chromat., 20, 89

Groll, H.P.A. (1933) Vapor-phase cracking. Industr. engng Chem., 25, 784

Heller, I. (1930) Cancer caused by coal tar and coal tar products. Occupational cancers. J. industr. Hyg., 12, 169

Hendricks, N.V., Liden, C.E., Berry, C.M., Lione, J.G. & Thorpe, J.J. (1959) Cancer of the scrotum in wax pressmen. Arch. industr. Hlth, 19, 524

Henry, S.A. (1946) Cancer of the scrotum in relation to occupation. London, New York, Toronto, Oxford University Press

Henry, S.A. (1947) Occupational cutaneous cancer attributable to certain chemicals in industry. Brit. med. Bull., 4, 389

Holmes, J.G., Kipling, M.D. & Waterhouse, J.A.H. (1970) Subsequent malignancies in men with scrotal epithelioma. Lancet, ii, 214

Howard, J.W., Teague, R.T., White, R.H. & Fry, B.E. (1966) Extraction and estimation of polycyclic aromatic hydrocarbons in smoked foods. I. General method. J. Ass. off. analyt. Chem., 9, 595

Howard, J.W., Fazio, T., White, R.H. & Klineck, B.A. (1968) Extraction and estimation of polycyclic aromatic hydrocarbons in total diet composites. J. Ass. off. analyt. Chem., 51, 122

Hueper, W.C. & Cahnmann, H.J. (1958) Carcinogenic bioassay of benzo(a)pyrene-free fractions of American shale oils. Arch. Path., 65, 608

Ingalls, T.H. (1950) Incidence of cancer in the carbon black industry. Arch. industr. Hyg., 1, 662

International Agency for Research on Cancer (1971) Standardization of sampling and analytical procedures for estimation of polynuclear aromatic hydrocarbons in the environment. IARC internal techn. Rep., No. 71/002

Jenkins, W.D. (1948) Dermatoses among gas and tar workers. Bristol, John Wright, p. 5

Jentoft, R.E. & Gouw, T.H. (1968) Separation of polycyclic aromatic hydrocarbons by high resolution liquid-liquid chromatography. Analyt. Chem., 40, 1787

Kawai, M., Amamoto, H. & Harada, K. (1967) Epidemiologic study of occupational lung cancer. Arch. environ. Hlth, 14, 859

Kennaway, E.L. (1925) Experiments on cancer-producing substances. Brit. med. J., ii, 1

Kennaway, E.L. & Hieger, I. (1930) Carcinogenic substances and their fluorescence spectra. Brit. med. J., i, 1044

Kennaway, E.L. & Kennaway, N.M. (1947) A further study of the incidence of cancer of the lung and larynx. Brit. J. Cancer, 1, 260

Kipling, M.D. (1968) Oil and the skin (Annual report of HM Chief Inspector of Factories, 1967), London, HMSO, p. 105

Kotin, P. & Falk, H.L. (1959) The role and action of environmental agents in the pathogenesis of lung cancer. I. Air pollutants. Cancer, 12, 147

Kuroda, S. & Kawahata, K. (1936) Über die gewerbliche Entstehung des Lungenkrebses bei Generatorgasarbeitern. Z. Krebsforsch., 45, 36

Lawther, P.J., Commins, B.T. & Waller, R.E. (1965) A study of the concentrations of polycyclic aromatic hydrocarbons in gas works retort houses. Brit. J. industr. Med., 22, 13

Leitch, A. (1922) Paraffin cancer and its experimental production. Brit. med. J., ii, 1104

Lenson, N. (1956) Multiple cutaneous carcinoma after creosote exposure. *New Engl. J. Med.*, *254*, 520

Liebe, G. (1892) Über den Theer- oder Paraffinkrebs. *Med. Jahrb.*, *236*, 65

Lijinsky, W., Saffiotti, U. & Shubik, P. (1956) A study of the chemical constitution and carcinogenic action of creosote oil. *J. nat. Cancer Inst.*, *18*, 687

Lloyd, J.W. (1971) Long-term mortality study of steel-workers. V. Respiratory cancer in coke plant workers. *J. occup. Med.*, *13*, 53

Medical Research Council (1968) *The carcinogenic action of mineral oils, a chemical and biological study. Special Report Series No. 306*, London, HMSO

Murray, J.A. (1921) Experimental tar cancer in mice. *Brit. med. J.*, *2*, 795

Manouvriez, A. (1876) Maladies et hygiène des ouvriers, travaillant à la fabrication des agglomérés de houille et de brai. *Ann. Hyg. publ. (Paris)*, *45*, 459

Nau, C.A., Neal, J. & Stembridge, V. (1958a) A study of the physiological effects of carbon black. I. Ingestion. *Arch. industr. Hlth*, *17*, 21

Nau, C.A., Neal, J. & Stembridge, V. (1958b) A study of the physiological effects of carbon black. II. Skin contact. *Arch. industr. Hlth*, *17*, 511

O'Donovan, W.J. (1921) Carcinoma cutis in an anthracene factory. *Brit. J. Derm.*, *33*, 291

O'Donovan, W.J. (1928) *Cancer of the skin due to occupation.* In: *Report of the International Conference on Cancer, London*, Bristol, John Wright, p. 293

Passey, R.D. (1922) Experimental soot cancer. *Brit. med. J.*, *ii*, 1112

Pott, P. (1775) *Cancer scroti.* In: *Chirurgical observations.* London, Hawes, Clarke & Collins, p. 63

Ross, P. (1948) Occupational skin lesions due to pitch and tar. *Brit. med. J.*, *ii*, 369

Sawicki, E. (1962) Analysis for airborne particulate hydrocarbons: their relative proportions as affected by different types of pollution. Nat. Cancer Inst. Monogr., 9, 201

Sawicki, E. (1964) The separation and analysis of polynuclear aromatic hydrocarbons present in the human environment. I-III. Chemist-Analyst, 53, 24, 56, 88

Sawicki, E., Corey, R.C., Dooley, A.E., Gisclard, J.B., Monkman, J.L., Neligan, R.E. & Ripperton, L.A. (1970) Tentative method of analysis for polynuclear aromatic hydrocarbon content of atmospheric particulate matter. Hlth lab. Sci., 7, Suppl., 31

Schaad, R.E. (1970) Chromatographie (karzinogener) polycyclischer aromatischer Kohlenwasserstoffe. Chromat. Rev., 13, 61

Schamberg, J.F. (1910) Cancer in tar workers. J. cutan. Dis., 28, 644

Shubik, P., Saffiotti, U., Lijinsky, W., Pietra, G., Rappaport, H., Toth, B., Raha, C.R., Tomatis, L., Feldman, R. & Ramahi, H. (1962) Studies on the toxicity of petroleum waxes. Toxicol. appl. Pharmacol., 4, 1

Smith, W.E., Sunderland, D.A. & Sugiura, K. (1951) Experimental analysis of the carcinogenic activity of certain petroleum products. Arch. industr. Hyg., 4, 299

Smith, W.M. (1970) Evaluation of coke oven emissions. Yb. amer. iron steel Inst., 163

Southam, A. (1928) Mule-spinners' cancer. In: Report of the International Conference on Cancer, London, Bristol, John Wright, p. 280

Stocks, P., Commins, B.T. & Aubrey, K.V. (1961) A study of polycyclic hydrocarbons and trace elements in smoke in Merseyside and other northern localities. Int. J. air wat. Pollut., 4, 141

Sulman, E. & Sulman, F. (1946) The carcinogenicity of wood soot from the chimney of a smoked sausage factory. Cancer Res., 6, 366

Tara, S. (1960) Noir de carbone (carbon black). *Rev. Path. gen.*, *60*, 643

Thony, C. & Thony, J. (1970) *Enquête épidémiologique sur le cancer des huiles de coupe.* In: *Proceedings of the 16th Congress of the Permanent Commission and International Association on Occupational Health, Tokyo, 1969*, Tokyo, Japan Industrial Safety Association, p. 655

Tsutsui, H. (1918) Über das künstlich erzeugte Cancroid bei der Maus. *Gann*, *12*, 17

Twort, C.C. & Fulton, J.S. (1930) Further experiments on the carcinogenicity of synthetic tars and their fractions. *J. Path. Bact.*, *32*, 119

Twort, C.C. & Twort, J.M. (1931) The carcinogenic potency of mineral oils. *J. industr. Hyg.*, *13*, 204

UICC (1970) *The quantification of environmental carcinogens* (UICC Technical Report Series, Vol. 4)

van Langermeersch, A. (1968) Identification et dosage des hydrocarbures cancérigènes. *Chimie Analytique*, *50*, 3

Volkmann, R. (1875) *Über Theer- Paraffin- und Russkrebs, (Schornsteinfegerkrebs).* In: *Beiträge zur Chirurgie*, Leipzig, Breitkopf und Hartel

Von Haam, E. & Mallette, F.S. (1952) Studies on toxicity and skin effects of compounds used in rubber and plastics industries: carcinogenicity of carbon blacks extracts. *Arch. industr. Hyg.*, *6*, 237

deVries, W.M. (1928) *Pitch cancer in the Netherlands.* In: *Report of the International Conference on Cancer*, London, Bristol, John Wright, p. 290

Waller, R.E. & Commins, B.T. (1967) Studies of the smoke and polycyclic aromatic hydrocarbon content of the air in large urban areas. *Environ. Res.*, *1*, 295

Waterhouse, J.A.H. (1971) Cutting oils and cancer. *Ann. occup. Hyg.*, *14*, 161

World Health Organization (1970) *European standards for drinking-water*, 2nd ed., Copenhagen

Wynder, E.L. & Hoffmann, D. (1967) Tobacco and tobacco smoke: Studies in experimental carcinogenesis, London, New York, Academic Press

Yamagiwa, K. & Ichikawa, K. (1915) Über die künstliche Erzeugung von Papillom. V. jap. path. Ges., 5, 142

POLYCYCLIC AROMATIC HYDROCARBONS

BENZ(a)ANTHRACENE*

1. Chemical and Physical Data

1.1 Synonyms

Chem. Abstr. No.: 56-55-3

1,2-Benzanthracene; 2,3-Benzphenanthrene;
2,3-Benzophenanthrene; Benzo(b)phenanthrene;
Tetraphene; Naphthanthracene; Benzanthrene; BA

1.2 Chemical formula and molecular weight

$C_{18}H_{12}$ Mol. wt: 228.28

1.3 Chemical and physical properties of the pure substance

(a) Description: Colourless leaflets or plates with yellowish green (to violet) fluorescence. General description in Beilsteins handbook, and in Clar (1964).

(b) Boiling-point: 400°C

(c) Melting-point: 159-161°C (from alcohol or glacial acetic acid)

(d) Absorption spectroscopy: The ultra-violet absorption spectrum is described by Sawicki et al. (1960a, b); by Carruthers & Douglas (1961), in pentane; by Borneff & Fischer (1963), in benzene; by Badger et al. (1965); and by Clar (1964). The fluorescence spectrum is given by Schoental & Scott (1949), in petroleum ether; by Sawicki et al. (1960a, b), in

---

* Considered by the Working Group in Lyon, December 1972.

pentane; and by Borneff & Fischer (1962), in benzene. The infra-red absorption spectrum is described by Fuson & Josien (1956) and in the API Research Project 44 (1960).

(e) <u>Identity and purity test</u>: Benz(a)anthracene (BA) forms a picrate with a melting-point of 141.5-142.5°C (red needles, from benzene or xylene) and a complex with 2,4,7-trinitrofluorenone (red needles, melting-point 223.6-224°C from alcohol) and with s-trinitrobenzene (orange needles, melting-point 162-163°C, 159.8-160.2°C from alcohol). The styphnate $C_{24}H_{15}N_3O_8$ melts at 153°C.

(f) <u>Solubility and/or volatility</u>: One litre of water dissolves 0.011 mg BA at 27°C (Davis et al., 1942). The substance is soluble in most organic solvents except alcohol. The distribution coefficients in the methanol-water/nitromethane system are given by Hoffmann & Wynder (1962a). BA is sublimable.

(g) <u>Chemical reactivity</u>: BA reacts as a diene in the Diels-Alder reaction (Jones et al., 1948; Tye et al., 1966). It adds maleic anhydride in the 7,12 position, and this reaction is suitable for separating BA from other non-reactive hydrocarbons. It is hydrogenated by sodium to the 7,12-dihydro compound, or under other conditions to the 1,2,3,4,7,12-hexahydro compound. Catalytic hydrogenation yields 8,9,10,11-tetrahydrobenzanthracene. Oxidation with sodium dichromate in glacial acetic acid gives the 7,12-quinone (Clar, 1964). In glacial acetic acid BA is quantitatively hydrogenated at 25°C with Adams catalyst to octadecahydrobenzanthracene (Jarman, 1971). There is no special position for electrophilic substitution.

2. Use and Occurrence

(a) Analytical methods

Several chromatographic procedures for the separation of BA from other substances and for its spectroscopic determination have been published and are extensively reviewed by Sawicki (1964) and by Schaad (1970). They include paper chromatography; column chromatography, used for detection in air (Sawicki et al., 1970); thin-layer chromatography (Hood & Winefordner, 1968); gas chromatography, used for detection in air (Chakraborty & Long, 1967) and for detection in soot (Searl et al., 1970); gel chromatography (Edstrom & Petro, 1968); ultra-violet absorption spectroscopy (Sawicki et al., 1970; Searl et al., 1970); fluorescence spectroscopy and low temperature fluorescence (Hood & Winefordner, 1968). References to analytical methods used for detection in various other media such as air, cigarette smoke, food, etc. can be found in the section on "Occurrence".

(b) Occurrence

Exhaust: Hoffmann & Wynder (1962a,b) isolated 61.7 mg/kg exhaust tar from gasoline engine exhaust and 4.2 µg from automobile exhaust gas after a one minute run. Two cyclic diesel engines run under various conditions produced 2.3-15 µg/m^3 of exhaust (Reckner et al., 1965).

Air: Detailed studies of air pollution in various cities in Europe, USA and Australia showed that in general concentrations depended on geographic location, the presence of nearby sources of pollution such as traffic, highways or industries, and on the season. Summer values ranged from 1.6 µg/1000 m^3 in Siena (Bosco et al., 1967) to 136 µg/1000 m^3 in Pittsburgh

(DeMaio & Corn, 1966), and winter values ranged from 94 µg/1000 m^3 in Siena (Bosco et al., 1967) to 361 µg/1000 m^3 in Bochum (Grimmer, 1966). In Sydney, Cincinnati and Detroit concentrations ranging from 0.6-13.7 µg/1000 m^3 (Cleary, 1963; Conlee et al., 1967; Colucci & Begeman, 1965) were found depending on the traffic situation. Examination of particulates or extracts gave the following results: 43-280 µg/g of organic atmospheric particulate matter in six American cities (Epstein et al., 1966); 9.6 (winter value) to 34.7 µg/g (summer value) in Sydney (Cleary & Sullivan, 1965); up to 555.5 µg/g of dust in three German cities (Hettche, 1965); 16-21 µg/kg of dust from roads near a highway (Borneff & Kunte, 1965); and 21.3-59 µg/kg in tunnel dust extracts (Grimmer & Hildebrandt, 1965a).

<u>Cigarette smoke</u>: Concentrations ranging from 1.2-14 µg were found in the smoke condensate of 100 cigarettes (Bonnet & Neukomm, 1956; Chakraborty et al., 1971; Cook, 1961; Kiryu & Kuratsune, 1966; Lindsey, 1959; Scassellati-Sforzolini et al., 1967; Wynder & Hoffmann, 1963), and in cigarette smoke condensate 0.03 µg/g (Wynder & Hoffmann, 1959) and 4.6 µg/g (Elmenhorst & Grimmer, 1968).

<u>Pyrolysis</u>: Up to 2.7 mg/kg BA are formed by the pyrolysis of a number of the major constituents of cured tobacco at 650°C (Gilbert & Lindsey, 1957); up to 168 mg/kg by the pyrolysis of carbohydrates, amino acids and fatty acids at 700°C and up to 0.5 mg/kg at 500°C (Masuda et al., 1967).

<u>Occupational exposure</u>: Kreyberg (1959) isolated concentrations ranging from 800-14 000 µg/1000 m^3 in the air of two gas works and one electrical plant. In air

polluted by coal-tar pitch 0.7 mg/1000 m^3 were detected, and up to 1300 mg/1000 m^3 were found in industrial effluents (Sawicki et al., 1965).

BA is found in different kinds of soot and smoke: e.g., in the soot of pre-mixed acetylene-oxygen flames (Long & Tompkins, 1967) and in wood smoke (Rhee & Bratzler, 1968). In flue gases from various coal-fired installations 44-5700 µg/1000 m^3 have been found (Diehl et al., 1967), and the emission levels of BA from heat generation sources (coal) ranged from 19-3900 µg/10^6 Btu[1] of heat input. The emission levels from incineration and open burning (of municipal refuse, automobile tyres, etc.) ranged from 0.09-0.26 µg/g of particulate matter for a municipal incinerator, 5-210 µg/g for a commercial incinerator, and 25-560 µg/g in open burning (Hangebrauck et al., 1964).

In addition, BA occurs in the aromatic fraction of a clarified oil (Dietz et al., 1956); in commercial solvents (hexane, 280 µg/kg; benzene, 1.8 µg/kg) (Lijinsky & Raha, 1961) and waxes (29 µg/kg) (Howard & Haenni, 1963); in Kuwait mineral oil (Carruthers & Douglas, 1961); in petrolatum (0.9 mg/kg), creosote (up to 2940 mg/kg) and coal-tar (up to 6980 mg/kg) (Lijinsky et al., 1963); and in petroleum asphalt (up to 35 mg/kg) and coal-tar pitch (up to 12 500 mg/kg) (Wallcave et al., 1971).

Soil and water: Fritz & Engst (1971) found 390 µg/kg BA in soil around an industrial centre, 1500 µg/kg near traffic highways, and up to 2500 mg/kg in soil polluted by coal-tar pitch. In soil samples from different areas in Germany (forest, woodland and sand) concentrations of BA

---

[1] British thermal unit

ranged from 5-20 µg/kg (Borneff & Kunte, 1963; Fritz & Engst, 1971).

In samples of drinking-water BA has been identified in concentrations of 1-23.2 µg/m^3 (Borneff & Kunte, 1964). In several samples of effluents a wide range of concentrations (25-10 360 µg/m^3) has been found, possibly due to industrial effluents or to water with bituminous contamination. In surface water 4.3-185 µg/m^3 have been found (Borneff & Kunte, 1964, 1965); and as much as 31.4 mg/m^3 were determined in sewage water from household, trade, road and industrial sources (Borneff & Kunte, 1967).

Food: In meat or fish the amount of BA present depends on the method of cooking: time of exposure, distance from the heat source and whether or not the melted fat is allowed to drop into the heat source. In broiled meat and sausages, concentrations ranged from 0.2-1.1 µg/kg (Grimmer & Hildebrandt, 1967a); in smoked ham and sausages 0.4-9.6 µg/kg were found (Howard et al., 1966a; Malanoski et al., 1968); while heavily smoked ham contained up to 12 µg/kg (Toth, 1971). In charcoal-broiled or -barbecued meat, concentrations ranged from 1.4-31 µg/kg (Fábián, 1968; Lijinsky & Shubik, 1964, 1965a; Lijinsky & Ross, 1967; Malanoski et al., 1968). In gas-broiled fish, up to 2.9 µg/kg were found (Masuda et al., 1966a). The concentrations in smoked fish ranged from 0.02-2.8 µg/kg (Grimmer & Hildebrandt, 1967a; Howard et al., 1966a; Lijinsky & Shubik, 1965b), while Masuda & Kuratsune (1971) detected up to 189 µg/kg. BA was also found in the smoke of charcoal-broiled bacon (Elmenhorst & Dontenwill, 1967) and of gas- and electric-broiled fish (Masuda et al., 1966a).

In vegetables the following amounts of BA were found: salad, 4.6-15.4 µg/kg; tomatoes, 0.3 µg/kg; spinach, 16.1 µg/kg; and kale, 43.6-230 µg/kg (Grimmer & Hildebrandt, 1965c; Hettche, 1971). Cereals were contaminated to variable degrees (0.4-6.8 µg/kg, depending on their source) (Grimmer & Hildebrandt, 1965b), and this amount is transferred to flour and bread (Fritz, 1968c).

In different kinds of crude and refined vegetable oils and fats, values between 0.5 and 13.5 µg/kg have been found, while in samples of crude coconut oil up to 98 µg/kg and in crude coconut fat up to 125 µg/kg have been detected (Biernoth & Rost, 1967, 1968; Borneff & Fábián, 1966; Fábián, 1968; Grimmer & Hildebrandt, 1967b). The BA content of these oils and fats decreased slightly with frying (Berner & Biernoth, 1969; Fritz, 1968d). Howard et al. (1966b) found 0.8-1.1 µg/kg in samples of refined vegetable oils, and Ciusa et al. (1965) detected BA in pressed or rectified olive oil. In margarine and mayonnaise 1.4-29.5 µg/kg have been found (Fábián, 1968, 1969; Fritz, 1968a).

In roasted coffee and soluble coffee powders, concentrations ranging from 0.5-14.2 µg/kg are reported (Fritz, 1968b, 1969; Kuratsune & Hueper, 1960), and in malt coffee up to 43 µg/kg were found (Fritz, 1968b). Peanuts roasted to two different degrees contained up to 0.95 µg/kg (Ballschmieter, 1969). In baker's dry yeast, Grimmer & Wilhelm (1969) detected 2.5-93.5 µg/kg, while dietetic yeasts or feed yeasts grown on mineral oil show a lower content. Masuda et al. (1966b) found 0.04-0.08 µg/l in two kinds of whisky.

Other material: In algae (chlorella vulgaris) about 7.5 µg/kg were found (Borneff et al., 1968).

3. Biological Data Relevant to the Evaluation of Carcinogenic Risk to Man

3.1 Carcinogenicity and related studies in animals

(a) <u>Oral administration</u>

<u>Mouse</u>: A single administration of 0.5 mg BA in mineral oil by stomach tube produced no tumours among 13 mice observed for 16 months. Eight or 16 administrations at three- to seven-day intervals produced a papilloma of the forestomach in 2/27 mice, whereas no tumours appeared among 16 controls given mineral oil only (Bock & King, 1959).

A total of 59 B6AF1/J mice received 15 treatments (over a period of five weeks) of 1.5 mg BA as a 3% solution in methocelaerosol OF by stomach tube starting at seven to eight days of age. In total, 56 developed lung adenomas, 38 had hepatomas and two had papillomas of the forestomach. Of 20 animals with median age at death of 547-600 days, all had hepatomas. Ten treatments with the same dose of 3-methylcholanthrene produced hepatomas in 49%, lung adenomas in 100% and forestomach papillomas in 63% of mice. In a group of 20 mice given only two treatments of BA three days apart, and dying at a median age of 547-600 days, 16 had hepatomas and 17 had lung adenomas. Among 59 controls, two had hepatomas, 10 had lung adenomas and none had tumours of the gastrointestinal tract (Klein, 1963).

(b) <u>Skin application</u>

<u>Mouse</u>: Kennaway (1930) painted 50 mice with BA in benzene at unspecified concentration and frequency; one regressing papilloma appeared. One epithelioma appeared

among 80 stock mice receiving a 2% solution in benzene, at unspecified intervals, of which only 23 were alive after six months (Barry et al., 1935). Similarly, one papilloma occurred among 20 mice painted twice weekly for 68 weeks with a 0.4% solution in mineral oil (Hill et al., 1951). In a more recent experiment, C3H/He mice were painted thrice weekly with different concentrations of BA either in toluene or in n-dodecane. With toluene, tumours (mostly malignant) were produced in mice as follows: at a 0.002% concentration, 0/32; at 0.02% concentration, 1/18; at 0.2% concentration, 3/32; at 1% concentration, 8/29. When BA in dodecane was used, incidences were: at 0.0002% concentration, 4/31; at 0.002% concentration, 8/21; at 0.02% concentration, 4/20; at 0.2% concentration, 11/21; at 1% concentration, 17/22. With the exception of some animals in the latter group, all tumours appeared after 50 weeks of treatment (Bingham & Falk, 1969). When comparing effective doses of BA and benzo(a)pyrene in dodecane, a 0.05% solution of benzo(a)pyrene produced tumours in 10/10 animals in 11 weeks; whereas a 0.2% solution of BA produced tumours in 11/21 animals with an average latent period of 61 weeks, and a 1% solution produced tumours in 17/22 with an average latent period of 42 weeks.

Graffi et al. (1953) obtained a 100% tumour incidence among 17 surviving mice at nine months, and 18 papillomas among nine surviving mice at 12 months after alternate, once-weekly application to 75 mice of 0.05% BA in acetone and 5% croton oil in mineral oil; controls receiving croton oil alone showed only 1/13 tumours. The ability of BA to initiate skin carcinogenesis in mice was first demonstrated by Roe & Salaman (1955). Ten applications of BA in acetone to 20 mice over a period of five weeks (total dose, 6 mg), followed by weekly applications of croton oil, produced a total of 21 skin tumours in 7/18 mice within 21 weeks. The treatment with BA alone did not produce tumours. This result was confirmed by Hadler et al. (1959) using a single application of 0.9 µg BA in acetone followed by croton oil (8/20 mice developed a total of 14 tumours) and by Van Duuren (1970) using a single application of 1 mg BA in benzene followed by phorbol myristate acetate (10/20 mice developed a total of 17 papillomas). In both these studies, controls given a single treatment with BA developed no tumours.

Rat: Twenty-five Donryru rats were painted daily for five months with a saturated solution of BA in acetone; no tumours developed in nine rats surviving for 18 months (Tawfic, 1965).

Hamster: Ten Syrian golden hamsters received bi-weekly paintings with 0.5% BA in mineral oil for 10 weeks. Six animals were surviving at 50 weeks, and the last animal died at 85 weeks; no tumours were recorded (Shubik et al., 1960).

(c) Subcutaneous and/or intramuscular administration

Mouse: A single injection of 5 mg BA in tricaprylin induced sarcomas in eight of 50 C57BL mice (Steiner & Falk, 1951). On the other hand, the simultaneous administration of 5 mg BA and 20 µg dibenz(a,h)anthracene resulted in an inhibition of tumour yield to about half the sum of the individual tumour yields (Steiner & Falk, 1951).

One dose-response study with BA in tricaprylin injected to C57BL mice led to the following incidence of mice with tumours per survivors at nine months: with 0.05 mg, 5/43; with 0.2 mg, 11/43; with 1.0 mg, 15/31; with 5.0 mg, 49/145; with 10.0 mg, 5/16 (Steiner & Edgcomb, 1952). Subcutaneous injection of BA in arachis oil (10 weekly injections of 1 mg) produced sarcomas in 14/20 C57BL mice in 146-179 days (Boyland & Sims, 1967).

Newborn mouse: Single injections of 50 µg BA in 1% aqueous gelatine to newborn and two- to eight-day old BALB/c mice induced pulmonary adenomas or adenocarcinomas, with more tumours occurring in newborn mice (Roe et al., 1963).

Rat: Twenty rats received a s.c. injection of 1.9 mg BA in tricaprylin; all were alive after four months and nine after 14.5 months when the experiment was terminated. No tumours were recorded (Miller & Miller, 1963).

(d) Other experimental systems

Intravenous injection: Twenty-nine female Sprague-Dawley rats received three injections of 2 mg BA (approximately 13 mg/kg) at intervals of three days, starting at 50 days of age. The animals were killed after 98 days and no mammary tumours were found (Pataki & Huggins, 1969).

Bladder implantation: Experiments using crushed paraffin wax as a vehicle were carried out by Clayson et al. (1968). With this technique about 2 mg BA induced 17 carcinomas and one papilloma in the bladders of 52 mice surviving 40 or more weeks. The incidence of tumours in the controls was 3.8%.

Homburger & Treger (1970) observed two tumours in 48 surviving C57/BL/6 J mice after a single s.c. injection of 500 µg BA in 0.1 ml tricaprylin without transfer of injection site. The yield of tumours in experiments with transfer of injection site after eight to 24 weeks was considerably increased.

3.2 Other relevant biological data

Boyland & Sims (1965) and Sims (1970) found four main metabolites when BA was incubated with liver homogenates from rats. Two of them, 4-hydroxybenzanthracene and 5,6-dihydro-5,6-dihydroxybenz(a)anthracene were characterized by direct comparison with authentic compounds, and the other two metabolites are probably 3-hydroxybenz(a)anthracene and 8,9-dihydro-8,9-dihydroxybenz(a)anthracene. Quantitative estimates of the products were obtained by radioactivity measurements.

K-region epoxide and cis-dihydrodiol derivatives of BA have been found to be more active in the production of transformation in hamster embryo cells and ventral prostate cells than BA itself or the corresponding K-region phenol (Grover et al., 1971).

3.3 Observations in man

None were available to the Working Group.

4. Comments on Data Reported and Evaluation

4.1 Animal data

BA given by several routes of administration has proved to be carcinogenic in the mouse. It produced hepatomas and lung adenomas following repeated oral administration to young mice. In a parallel experiment with methylcholanthrene, the carcinogenic effect upon the liver and lung was similar for the two compounds at the same dose level. In the same experiment, BA did not produce tumours of the gastrointestinal tract, whereas methylcholanthrene induced them consistently.

BA is a complete carcinogen for the mouse skin. The fact that the tumour yield was higher when using a dodecane solution than with toluene is related to the co-carcinogenic effect of dodecane. Benzo(a)pyrene given at a lower dose level produced more skin tumours with a shorter latency period than did BA. BA is also an initiator of skin carcinogenesis in mice.

BA produced tumours in mice following s.c. injections. Fifty µg BA was the lowest dose tested, and it was effective in newborn and in adult animals. It produced bladder tumours in mice following implantation.

It has not been adequately tested in other species.

4.2 Human data

No case reports or epidemiological studies on the significance of BA exposure to man are available. However, coal-tar and other materials which are known to be carcinogenic to man may contain BA. The substance has also been detected in other environmental situations. The possible contribution of polycyclic aromatic hydrocarbons from some environmental sources to the overall carcinogenic risk to man is discussed in the preamble.

5. References

API Research Project 44 (1960) Selected Infrared Spectral Data, Vol. VI, No. 2236

Badger, G.M., Donnelly, J.K. & Spotswood, T.M. (1965) The formation of aromatic hydrocarbons at high temperatures. XXIV. The pyrolysis of some tobacco constituents. Aust. J. Chem., 18, 1249

Ballschmieter, H.M.B. (1969) Über polycyclische aromatische Kohlenwasserstoffe in gerösteten Erdnüssen. Fette, Seifen, Anstrichmittel, 71, 521

Barry, G., Cook, J.W., Haslewood, G.A.D., Hewett, C.L., Hieger, I. & Kennaway, E.L. (1935) The production of cancer by pure hydrocarbons. Part III. Proc. roy. Soc. B, 117, 318

Beilsteins Handbuch, der Organischen Chemie, 5, 718; 5, II, 628; 5, III, 2375

Berner, G. & Biernoth, G. (1969) Über den Gehalt erhitzter Öle und Fette an polycyclischen aromatischen Kohlenwasserstoffen. Z. Lebensmitt.-Untersuch., 140, 330

Biernoth, G. & Rost, H.E. (1967) The occurrence of polycyclic aromatic hydrocarbons in coconut oil and their removal. Chem. and Ind., 2002

Biernoth, G. & Rost, H.E. (1968) Vorkommen polycyclischer aromatischer Kohlenwasserstoffe in Speiseölen und deren Entfernung. Arch. Hyg. (Muenchen), 152, 238

Bingham, E. & Falk, H.L. (1969) Environmental carcinogens. The modifying effect of cocarcinogens on the threshold response. Arch. environ. Hlth, 19, 779

Bock, F.G. & King, D.W. (1959) A study of the sensitivity of the mouse forestomach toward certain polycyclic hydrocarbons. J. nat. Cancer Inst., 23, 833

Bonnet, J. & Neukomm, S. (1956) Sur la composition chimique de la fumée du tabac. I. Analyse de la fraction neutre. Helv. chim. Acta, 39, 1724

Borneff, J. & Fábián, B. (1966) Kanzerogene Substanzen in Speisefett und -öl. Arch. Hyg. (Muenchen), 150, 485

Borneff, J. & Fischer, R. (1962) Kanzerogene Substanzen in Wasser und Boden. XI. Polyzyklische, aromatische Kohlenwasserstoffe in Walderde. Arch. Hyg. (Muenchen), 146, 430

Borneff, J. & Kunte, H. (1963) Kanzerogene Substanzen in Wasser und Boden. XIV. Weitere Untersuchungen über polyzyklische aromatische Kohlenwasserstoffe in Erdproben. Arch. Hyg. (Muenchen), 147, 401

Borneff, J. & Kunte, H. (1964) Kanzerogene Substanzen in Wasser und Boden. XVI. Nachweis von polyzyklischen Aromaten in Wasserproben durch direkte Extraktion. Arch. Hyg. (Muenchen), 148, 585

Borneff, J. & Kunte, H. (1965) Kanzerogene Substanzen in Wasser und Boden. XVII. Über die Herkunft und Bewertung der polyzyklischen, aromatischen Kohlenwasserstoffe im wasser. Arch. Hyg. (Muenchen), 149, 226

Borneff, J. & Kunte, H. (1967) Kanzerogene Substanzen in Wasser und Boden. XIX. Wirkung der Abwasserreinigung auf polyzyklische Aromaten. Arch. Hyg. (Muenchen), 151, 202

Borneff, J., Selenka, F., Kunte, H. & Maximos, A. (1968) Experimental studies on the formation of polycyclic aromatic hydrocarbons in plants. Environ. Res., 2, 22

Bosco, G., Barsini, G. & Grella, A. (1967) Nuove indagini sulla presenza di idrocarburi policiclici aromatici nel pulviscolo atmosferico del centro storico della citta di Siena. Arch. environ. Hlth, 14, 285

Boyland, E. & Sims, P. (1965) The metabolism of benz(a)anthracene and dibenz(a,h)anthracene and their 5,6-epoxy-5,6-dihydro derivatives by rat-liver homogenates. Biochem. J., 97, 7

Boyland E. & Sims, P. (1967) The carcinogenic activities in mice of compounds related to benz(a)anthracene. Int. J. Cancer, 2, 500

Carruthers, W. & Douglas, A.G. (1961) 1,2-Benzanthracene derivatives in a Kuwait mineral oil. Nature (Lond.), 192 256

Chakraborty, B.B. & Long, R. (1967) Gas chromatographic analysis of polycyclic aromatic hydrocarbons in soot samples. Environ. Sci. Technol., 1, 828

Chakraborty, B.B., **Kilburn, K.D.** & Thornton, R.E. (1971) Reduction in the concentration of aromatic polycyclic hydrocarbons in cigarette smoke. Chem. and Ind., 672

Ciusa, W., Nebbia, G., Buccelli, A. & Volpones, E. (1965) Ricerche sopra gli idrocarburi policiclici aromatici presenti negli olii di oliva. Riv. ital. Sost. grasse, 42, 175

Clar, E. (1964) Polycyclic Hydrocarbons, Vol. 1, London, New York, Academic Press; Berlin, Göttingen, Heidelberg, Springer-Verlag, p.307

Clayson, D.B., Pringle, J.A.S., Bonser, G.M. & Wood, M. (1968) The technique of bladder implantation: further results and an assessment. Brit. J. Cancer, 22, 825

Cleary, G.J. (1963) Measurement of polycyclic aromatic hydrocarbons in the air of Sydney using very long alumina columns for separation. Int. J. air wat. Pollut., 7, 753

Cleary, G.J. & Sullivan, J.L. (1965) Pollution by polycyclic aromatic hydrocarbons in the city of Sydney. Med. J. Aust., 1, 758

Colucci, J.M. & Begeman, C.R. (1965) The automotive contribution to air-borne polynuclear aromatic hydrocarbons in Detroit. J. air Pollut. Control Ass., 15, 113

Conlee, C.J., Kenline, P.A., Cummins, R.L. & Konopinski, V.J. (1967) Motor vehicle exhaust at three selected sites. Arch. environ. Hlth, 14, 429

Cook, J.W. (1961) Tobacco smoke and lung cancer. The Royal Institute of Chemistry Lecture Series, No. 5

Davis, W.W., Krahl, M.E. & Clowes, G.H.A. (1942) Solubility of carcinogenic and related hydrocarbons in water. J. amer. chem. Soc., 64, 108

DeMaio, L. & Corn, M. (1966) Polynuclear aromatic hydrocarbons associated with particulates in Pittsburgh air. J. air. Pollut. Control Ass., 16, 67

Diehl, E.K., du Breuil, F. & Glenn, R.A. (1967) Polynuclear hydrocarbon emission from coal-fired installations. J. Engng. Power, 89, 276

Dietz, W.A., Dudenbostal, B.F. & Priestley, W. (1956) Analysis of high boiling petroleum fractions by ultra-violet spectrometry. Amer. chem. Soc., Div. petrol. Chem. Preprints, 1, 117

Edstrom, T. & Petro, B.A. (1968) Gel permeation chromatographic studies of polynuclear aromatic hydrocarbon materials. J. polymer Sci. C, 21, 171

Elmenhorst, H. & Dontenwill, W. (1967) Nachweis cancerogener Kohlenwasserstoffe im Rauch beim Grillen über Holzkohlenfeuer. Z. Krebsforsch., 70, 157

Elmenhorst, H. & Grimmer, G. (1968) Polycyclische Kohlenwasserstoffe aus Zigarettenrauchkondensat. Eine Methode zur Fraktionierung grosser Mengen für Tierversuche. Z. Krebsforsch., 71, 66

Epstein, S.S., Joshi, S., Andrea, J., Mantel, N., Sawicki, E., Stanley, T. & Tabor, E.C. (1966) Carcinogenicity of organic particulate pollutants in urban air after administration of trace quantities to neonatal mice. Nature (Lond.), 212, 1305

Fábián, B. (1968) Kanzerogene Substanzen in Speisefett und -öl. V. Untersuchungen an verschieden zubereiteten Bratwürsten. Arch. Hyg. (Muenchen), 152, 251

Fábián, B. (1969) Kanzerogene Substanzen in Speisefett und -öl. VI. Weitere Untersuchungen an Margerine und Schokolade. Arch. Hyg. (Muenchen), 153, 21

Fritz, W. (1968a) 3,4-Benzpyren und andere Polyaromaten in Margarine und Mayonnaise. Nahrung, 12, 495

Fritz, W. (1968b) Zur Bildung cancerogener Kohlenwasserstoffe bei der thermischen Behandlung von Lebensmitteln. II. Das Rösten von Bohnenkaffee und Kaffee-Ersatzstoffen. Nahrung, 12, 799

Fritz, W. (1968c) Zur Bildung cancerogener Kohlenwasserstoffe bei der thermischen Behandlung von Lebensmitteln. III. Das Backen von Brot und Biskuits. Nahrung, 12, 805

Fritz, W. (1968d) Zur Bildung cancerogener Kohlenwasserstoffe bei der thermischen Behandlung von Lebensmitteln. IV. Der Einfluss des Frittierens. Nahrung, 12, 809

Fritz, W. (1969) Zum Lösungsverhalten der Polyaromaten beim Kochen von Kaffee-Ersatzstoffen und Bohnenkaffee. Dtsch. Lebensmitt.-Rdsch., 65, 83

Fritz. W. & Engst, R. (1971) Zur umweltbedingten Kontamination von Lebensmitteln mit krebserzeugenden Kohlenwasserstoffen. Z. ges. Hyg., 17, 271

Fuson, N. & Josien, M.L. (1956) Infra-red spectra of polynuclear aromatic compounds. I. 1,2-Benzanthracene, the monomethyl-1,2-benzanthracenes and some dimethyl-1,2-benzanthracenes. J. amer. chem. Soc., 78, 3049

Gilbert, J.A.S. & Lindsey, A.J. (1957) The thermal decomposition of some tobacco constituents. Brit. J. Cancer, 11, 398

Graffi, A., Vlamynck, E., Hoffmann, F. & Schulz, I. (1953) Untersuchungen über die geschwulstauslösende Wirkung verschiedener chemischer Stoffe in der Kombination mit Crotonöl. Arch. Geschwulstforsch., 5, 110

Grimmer, G. (1966) Cancerogene Kohlenwasserstoffe in der Umgebung des Menschen. Erdöl Kohle-Erdgas-Petrochem., 19, 578

Grimmer, G. & Hildebrandt, A. (1965a) Kohlenwasserstoffe in der Umgebung des Menschen. I. Eine Methode zur simultanen Bestimmung von dreizehn polycyclischen Kohlenwasserstoffen. J. Chromat., 20, 89

Grimmer, G. & Hildebrandt, A. (1965b) Kohlenwasserstoffe in der Umgebung des Menschen. II. Der Gehalt polycyclischer Kohlenwasserstoffe in Brotgetreide verschiedener Standorte. Z. Krebsforsch., 67, 272

Grimmer, G. & Hildebrandt, A. (1965c) Kohlenwasserstoffe in der Umgebung des Menschen. III. Der Gehalt polycyclischer Kohlenwasserstoffe in verschiedenen Gemüsesorten und Salaten. Dtsch. Lebensmitt.-Rdsch., 61, 272

Grimmer, G. & Hildebrandt, A. (1967a) Kohlenwasserstoffe in der Umgebung des Menschen. V. Der Gehalt polycyclischer Kohlenwasserstoffe in Fleisch und Räucherwaren. Z. Krebsforsch., 69, 223

Grimmer, G. & Hildebrandt, A. (1967b) Content of polycyclic hydrocarbons in crude vegetable oils. Chem. and Ind., 2000

Grimmer, G. & Wilhelm, G. (1969) Der Gehalt von polycyclischen Kohlenwasserstoffen in europäischen Hefen. Dtsch. Lebensmitt.-Rdsch., 65, 229

Grover, P.L., Sims, P., Huberman, E., Marquardt, H., Kuroki, T. & Heidelberger, C. (1971) In vitro transformation of rodent cells by K-region derivatives of polycyclic hydrocarbons. Proc. nat. Acad. Sci. (Wash.), 68, 1098

Hadler, H.I., Darchun, V. & Lee, K. (1959) Initiation and promotion activity of certain polynuclear hydrocarbons. J. nat. Cancer Inst., 23, 1383

Hangebrauck, R.P., von Lehmden, D.J. & Meeker, J.E. (1964) Emissions of polynuclear hydrocarbons and other pollutants from heat-generation and incineration processes. J. air Pollut. Control Ass., 14, 267

Hartwell, J.L. (1951) Survey of compounds which have been tested for carcinogenic activity, Washington, D.C., Government Printing Office (Public Health Service Publication No. 149)

Hettche, H.O. (1965) The measurement of polycyclic aromatics in the atmosphere. Staub (Engl. Transl.), 25, 41

Hettche, H.O. (1971) Plant waxes as collectors of polycyclic aromatics in the air of residential areas. Staub (Engl. Transl.), 31, 34

Hill, W.T., Stanger, D.W., Pizzo, A., Riegel, B., Shubik, P. & Wartman, W.B. (1951) Inhibition of 9,10-dimethyl-1,2-benzanthracene skin carcinogenesis in mice by polycyclic hydrocarbons. Cancer Res., 11, 892

Hoffmann, D. & Wynder, E.L. (1962a) Analytical and biological studies on gasoline engine exhaust. Nat. Cancer Inst. Monogr., 9, 91

Hoffmann, D. & Wynder, E.L. (1962b) A study of air pollution carcinogenesis. II. The isolation and identification of polynuclear aromatic hydrocarbons from gasoline engine exhaust condensate. Cancer, 15, 93

Homburger, F. & Treger, A. (1970) Transplantation technique for acceleration of carcinogenesis by benz(a)anthracene or 3,4,9,10-dibenzpyrene /benzo(r,s,t)pentaphene/. J. nat. Cancer Inst., 44, 357

Hood, L.V. & Winefordner, J.D. (1968) Thin-layer separation and low-temperature luminescence measurement of mixtures of carcinogens. Analyt. Chim. Acta, 42, 199

Howard, J.W. & Haenni, E.O. (1963) The extraction and determination of polynuclear hydrocarbons in paraffin waxes. J. Ass. off. agric. Chem., 46, 933

Howard, J.W., Teague, R.T., White, R.H. & Fry, B.E. (1966a) Extraction and estimation of polycyclic aromatic hydrocarbons in smoked foods. I. General method. J. Ass. off. analyt. Chem., 49, 595

Howard, J.W., Turicchi, E.W., White, R.H. & Fazio, T. (1966b) Extraction and estimation of polycyclic aromatic hydrocarbons in vegetable oils. J. Ass. off. analyt. Chem., 49, 1236

Jarman, M. (1971) Total reduction of benz(a)anthracene: the preparation of octadecahydrobenz(a)anthracene. Chem. and Ind., 8, 228

Jones, R.N., Gogek, C.J. & Sharpe, R.W. (1948) The reaction of maleic anhydride with polynuclear aromatic hydrocarbons. Canad. J. Res., 26, 719

Kennaway, E.L. (1930) Further experiments on cancer-producing substances. Biochem. J., 24, 497

Kiryu, S. & Kuratsune, M. (1966) Polycyclic aromatic hydrocarbons in the cigarette tar produced by human smoking. Gann, 57, 317

Klein, M. (1963) Susceptibility of strain B6AF$_1$/J hybrid infant mice to tumorigenesis with 1,2-benzanthracene, deoxycholic acid, and 3-methylcholanthrene. Cancer Res., 23, 1701

Kreyberg, L. (1959) 3,4-Benzpyrene in industrial air pollution: some reflexions. Brit. J. Cancer, 13, 618

Kuratsune, M. & Hueper, W.C. (1960) Polycyclic aromatic hydrocarbons in roasted coffee. J. nat. Cancer Inst., 24, 463

Lijinsky, W. & Raha, C.R. (1961) Polycyclic aromatic hydrocarbons in commercial solvents. Toxicol. appl. Pharmacol., 3, 469

Lijinsky, W. & Ross, A.E. (1967) Production of carcinogenic polynuclear hydrocarbons in the cooking of food. Food cosmet. Toxicol., 5, 343

Lijinsky, W. & Shubik, P. (1964) Benzo(a)pyrene and other polynuclear hydrocarbons in charcoal-broiled meat. Science, 145, 53

Lijinsky, W. & Shubik, P. (1965a) Polynuclear hydrocarbon carcinogens in cooked meat and smoked food. Industr. Med. Surg., 34, 152

Lijinsky, W. & Shubik, P. (1965b) The detection of polycyclic aromatic hydrocarbons in liquid smoke and some foods. Toxicol. appl. Pharmacol., 7, 337

Lijinsky, W., Domsky, I., Mason, G., Ramahi, H.Y. & Safavi, T. (1963) The chromatographic determination of trace amounts of polynuclear hydrocarbons in petroleum, mineral oil and coal-tar. Analyt. Chem., 35, 952

Lindsey, A.J. (1959) The composition of cigarette smoke: studies on stubs and tips. Brit. J. Cancer, 13, 195

Long, R. & Tompkins, E.E. (1967) Formation of polycyclic aromatic hydrocarbons in pre-mixed acetylene-oxygen flames. Nature (Lond.), 213, 1011

Malanoski, A.J., Greenfield, E.L., Barnes, C.J., Worthington, J.M. & Joe, F.L. (1968) Survey of polycyclic aromatic hydrocarbons in smoked foods. J. Ass. off. analyt. Chem., 51, 114

Masuda, Y. & Kuratsune, M. (1971) Polycyclic aromatic hydrocarbons in smoked fish, "katsuobushi". Gann, 62, 27

Masuda, Y., Mori, K. & Kuratsune, M. (1966a) Polycyclic aromatic hydrocarbons in common Japanese foods. I. Broiled fish, roasted barley, shoyu and caramel. Gann, 57, 133

Masuda, Y., Mori, K., Hirohata, T. & Kuratsune, M. (1966b) Carcinogenesis in the esophagus. III. Polycyclic aromatic hydrocarbons and phenols in whisky. Gann, 57, 549

Masuda, Y., Mori, K. & Kuratsune, M. (1967) Polycyclic aromatic hydrocarbons formed by pyrolysis of carbohydrates, amino acids and fatty acids. Gann, 58, 69

Miller, J.A. & Miller, E.C. (1963) The carcinogenicities of fluoro derivatives of 10-methyl-1,2-benzanthracene. II. Substitution of the K-region and the 3-, 6-, and 7-positions. Cancer Res., 23, 229

Pataki, J. & Huggins, C. (1969) Molecular site of substituents of benz(a)anthracene related to carcinogenicity. Cancer Res., 29, 506

Reckner, L.R., Scott, W.E. & Biller, W.F. (1965) The composition and odor of diesel exhaust. Proc. amer. petrol. Inst., 45, 133

Rhee, K.S. & Bratzler, L.J. (1968) Polycyclic hydrocarbon composition of wood smoke. J. food Sci., 33, 626

Roe, F.J.C. & Salaman, M.H. (1955) Further studies on incomplete carcinogenesis: triethylene melamine (TEM), 1,2-benzanthracene and β-propiolactone as initiators of skin tumour formation in the mouse. Brit. J. Cancer, 9, 177

Roe, F.J.C., Mitchley, B.C.V. & Walters, M. (1963) Tests for carcinogenesis using newborn mice, 1,2-benzanthracene, 2-naphthylamine, 2-naphthylhydroxylamine and ethyl methane sulphonate. Brit. J. Cancer, 17, 255

Sawicki, E. (1964) The separation and analysis of polynuclear aromatic hydrocarbons present in the human environment. I-III. Chemist-Analyst, 53, 24, 56, 88

Sawicki, E., Elbert, W., Stanley, T.W., Hauser, T.R. & Fox, F.T. (1960a) Separation and characterization of polynuclear aromatic hydrocarbons in urban air-borne particulates. Analyt. Chem., 32, 810

Sawicki, E., Hauser, T.R. & Stanley, T.W. (1960b) Ultraviolet, visible and fluorescence spectral analysis of polynuclear hydrocarbons. Int. J. air Pollut., 2, 253

Sawicki, E., Meeker, J.E. & Morgan, M.J. (1965) The quantitative composition of air pollution source effluents in terms of aza heterocyclic compounds and polynuclear aromatic hydrocarbons. Int. J. air wat. Pollut., 9, 291

Sawicki, E., Corey, R.C., Dooley, A.E., Gisclard, J.B., Monkman, J.L., Neligan, R.E. & Ripperton, L.A. (1970) Tentative method of analysis for polynuclear aromatic hydrocarbon content of atmospheric particulate matter. Hlth lab. Sci., 7, Suppl., 31

Scassellati-Sforzolini, G., Pascasio, F., Mastrandrea, F. & Savino, A. (1967) Attività cancerigena del fumo di sigaretta. Quantificazione degli idrocarburi aromatici policiclici presenti nella porzione aspirata. Riv. ital. Igiene, 27, 175

Schaad, R. (1970) Chromatographie (karzinogener) polyzyclische aromatischer Kohlenwasserstoffe. Chromat. Rev., 13, 61

Schoental, R. & Scott, E.J.Y. (1949) Fluorescence spectra of polycyclic aromatic hydrocarbons in solution. J. chem. Soc., 1683

Searl, T.D., Cassidy, F.J., King, W.H. & Brown, R.A. (1970) An analytical method for polynuclear aromatic compounds in coke oven effluents by combined use of gas chromatography and ultraviolet absorption spectrometry. Analyt. Chem., 42, 954

Shubik, P., Pietra, G. & Della Porta, G. (1960) Studies of skin carcinogenesis in the Syrian golden hamster. Cancer Res., 20, 100

Sims, P. (1970) Qualitative and quantitative studies on the metabolism of a series of aromatic hydrocarbons by rat-liver preparations. Biochem. Pharmacol., 19, 795

Steiner, P.E. & Edgcomb, J.H. (1952) Carcinogenicity of 1,2-benzanthracene. Cancer Res., 12, 657

Steiner, P.E. & Falk, H.L. (1951) Summation and inhibition effects of weak and strong carcinogenic hydrocarbons: 1,2-benzanthracene, chrysene, 1,2,5,6-dibenzanthracene, and 20-methylcholanthrene. Cancer Res., 11, 56

Tawfic, H.N. (1965) Studies on ear-duct tumors in rats. II. Inhibitory effect of methylcholanthrene and 1,2-benzanthracene on tumor formation by 4-dimethyl-aminostilbene. Acta path. jap., 15, 255

Tóth, L. (1971) Polyzyklische Kohlenwasserstoffe in geräuchertem Schinken und Bauchspeck. Fleischwirtschaft, 7, 1069

Tye, R., Horton, A.W. & Rapien, I. (1966) Benzo(a)pyrene and other aromatic hydrocarbons extractable from bituminous coal. Amer. industr. Hyg. Ass. J., 27, 25

Van Duuren, B.L., Sivak, A., Goldschmidt, B.M., Katz, C. & Melchionne, S. (1970) Initiating activity of aromatic hydrocarbons in two-stage carcinogenesis. J. nat. Cancer Inst., 44, 1167

Wallcave, L., Garcia, H., Feldman, R., Lijinsky, W. & Shubik, P. (1971) Skin tumorigenesis in mice by petroleum asphalts and coal-tar pitches of known polynuclear aromatic hydrocarbon content. Toxicol. appl. Pharmacol., 18, 41

Wynder, E.L. & Hoffmann, D. (1959) A study of tobacco carcinogenesis. VII. The role of higher polycyclic hydrocarbons. Cancer, 12, 1079

Wynder, E.L. & Hoffmann, D. (1963) Ein experimenteller Beitrag zur Tabakrauch-kanzerogenese. Dtsch. med. Wschr., 88, 623

BENZO(b)FLUORANTHENE*

1. Chemical and Physical Data

1.1 Synonyms

Chem. Abstr. No.: 205-99-2

Chem. Abstr. Name: Benz(e)acephenanthrylene

2,3-Benzofluoranthene; 3,4-Benzofluoranthene; B(b)F

1.2 Chemical formula and molecular weight

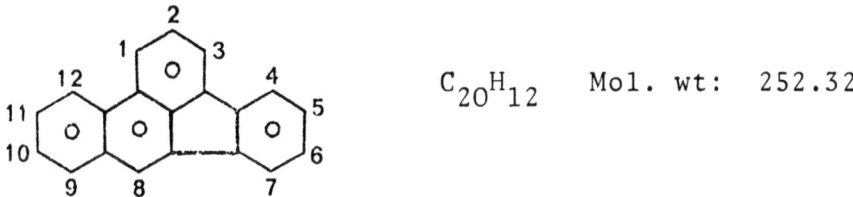

$C_{20}H_{12}$ Mol. wt: 252.32

1.3 Chemical and physical properties of the pure substance

(a) *Description*: Colourless needles from benzene, toluene or glacial acetic acid. General description in Beilsteins handbook, and in Clar (1964).

(b) *Melting-point*: 167-168°C

(c) *Absorption spectroscopy*: The ultra-violet absorption spectrum is described by Clar (1964), in ethanol; by Lyons (1959) and Hoffmann & Wynder (1962a), in cyclohexane; by Badger et al. (1965)

---

* Considered by the Working Group in Lyon, December 1972.

and Sawicki et al. (1960), in pentane. The ultraviolet absorption of benzo(b)fluoranthene (B(b)F), together with other polycyclic aromatic hydrocarbons in cyclohexane, was investigated by Scassellati-Sforzolini et al. (1967). The infra-red absorption spectrum of the solid and of B(b)F dissolved in CCl_4 or CS_2 were published by the API Research Project 44 (1961). The fluorescence and low-temperature fluorescence are described by Borneff & Fábián (1966). The maximum for fluorescence and the relative molar extinction are given by Sawicki et al. (1960) and by Sawicki (1969) who also discussed the influence of other factors. The fluorescence spectrum is also presented by Lyons (1959), and the nuclear magnetic resonance spectrum by Bartle et al. (1969).

(d) <u>Identity and purity test</u>: B(b)F forms a picrate with a melting-point of 156°C.

(e) <u>Solubility and/or volatility</u>: Hoffmann & Wynder (1962a) present partition coefficients for the 4:1 cyclohexane/methanolic water system and nitromethane/cyclohexane system as 14.7 and 1.94.

(f) <u>Chemical reactivity</u>: Data on π-electron energy were reported by Mallion (1970) and by Titz & Hochmann (1967).

2. Use and Occurrence

(a) Analytical methods

Several chromatographic procedures for the separation of B(b)F from other substances and for its spectroscopic determination have been published and are extensively reviewed by

Sawicki (1964) and by Schaad (1970). They include paper chromatography, used for detection in food (Howard & Teague, 1965); column chromatography; thin-layer chromatography (Matsushita & Suzuki, 1969; Short & Young, 1969), used for detection in air (Strömberg & Widmark, 1970; Matsushita et al., 1970); gas chromatography (Savino, 1968; Fryčka, 1972), used for detection in cigarette smoke (Davis, 1969), for detection in soot (Chakraborty & Long, 1967), and for detection in air (Brocco et al., 1970); gel chromatography (Edstrom & Petro, 1968); ultra-violet absorption spectroscopy (Strömberg & Widmark, 1970; Howard & Teague, 1965); fluorescence spectroscopy (Matsushita et al., 1970); and mass spectrometry (Strömberg & Widmark, 1970). References to analytical methods used for detection in various other media such as water, food, etc. can be found in the section on "Occurrence".

(b) Occurrence

Exhaust: Engines using gasoline as fuel produced 7.7 mg/1000 m^3 of exhaust (Del Vecchio et al., 1970), and 64 mg/kg of exhaust tar was isolated from first-run exhaust (Hoffmann & Wynder, 1962b). The output of automobiles' engines was 4.4 µg/minute run (Hoffmann & Wynder, 1962a). Engines using heavy liquified petroleum produced 0.9 mg/1000 m^3 of exhaust under idling conditions, but with normal working conditions this amount was markedly higher (3.9 mg/1000 m^3) (Del Vecchio et al., 1970). B(b)F was also present in petrol engine exhaust samples (Lyons, 1959).

Air: In the air of Sydney, concentrations ranged from 0.5-1.5 µg/1000 m^3 (Cleary, 1963) and in Siena from 0.25-5.3, the highest value being found in December (Bosco et al., 1967). Examination of particulates or extracts give the following results: 209-492 mg/kg in tar samples in the Detroit area (Colucci & Begeman, 1965); 15-62 mg/kg in dust from roads, and 0.16 mg/kg in dust from air (Borneff & Kunte, 1965).

Cigarette smoke: In the smoke condensate of 100 cigarettes, concentrations ranged between 0.1-2 µg (Kiryu & Kuratsune, 1966; Scassellati-Sforzolini et al., 1967; Wynder & Hoffmann, 1963), and approximately 3.7 µg B(b)F and benzo(j)fluoranthene[1] have been found (Ayres & Thornton, 1965). In smoke condensate 0.1 µg/kg have been found (Wynder & Hoffmann, 1959a).

Pyrolysis: B(b)F is formed by pyrolysis of anthracene at 700-850°C (Badger et al., 1964), of the tobacco constituents dotriacontane and stigmasterol at 700°C (Badger et al., 1965), and of carbohydrates, amino acids and fatty acids at 700°C (0.2-3 mg/kg) but not at 500°C (Masuda et al., 1967).

Occupational exposure: Kruber & Oberkobusch (1952) detected B(b)F in coal-tar, and soot samples showed an average concentration of 8.4 mg/kg (Fischer, 1970).

Soil and water: In woodland soil samples of different areas in Germany, concentrations of B(b)F and benzo(j)fluoranthene[1] ranged from 15-110 µg/kg (Borneff & Fischer, 1962; Borneff & Kunte, 1963). In the muddy deposits and in suspended matter of the Rhine river 1.8 and 1.3 mg/kg B(b)F and benzo(j)fluoranthene[1] were found (Borneff & Fischer, 1963). In drinking-water, concentrations ranged from 0.8-11.5 µg/m^3 B(b)F (Borneff & Kunte, 1964, 1969).

---

[1] The two substances could not be completely separated.

In river and lake water a wide range of concentrations has been found (39-9910 µg/m^3) depending on the industrial effluents in the water tested; while in surface water 3.7-156 µg/m^3 have been found in sewage water from household, industry and roads (Borneff & Kunte, 1967).

Food: In gas-broiled fish 0.1-1.2 µg/kg could be found (Masuda et al., 1966a), while smoked or dried fish could contain as much as 37 µg/kg (Masuda & Kuratsune, 1971). In heavily smoked ham or bacon 3.6-15.1 µg/kg were found (Toth, 1971), and in fresh sausages 0.4 µg/kg and in grilled or fried sausages 6.3 µg/kg have been detected (Fábián, 1968b). B(b)F has also been reported in the smoke of gas- or electric-broiled fish (Masuda et al., 1966a).

In olive oil, plant cooking fat, plant oil and coconut oil, concentrations ranged from 0.2-4 µg/kg (Borneff & Fábián, 1966; Fábián, 1968a), and in margarine from 2.6-14.5 µg/kg (Fábián, 1968a, 1969), the concentration being reduced by treatment with activated charcoal and steam. In fat, the concentration could be reduced by controlled laboratory heating (Borneff & Fábián, 1966) and in oils by frying (Fritz, 1968b).

Extremely black roasted coffee contained 1.2-2.1 µg/kg, and up to 3.0 µg/kg were found in malt coffee, substitute coffee and soluble coffee powder (Fritz, 1968a, 1969). In whisky 0.05 µg/l could be detected in only one out of 15 brands (Masuda et al., 1966b).

Other material: Gräf & Diehl (1966) found 62-374 µg/kg in leaves of various kinds of trees and in tobacco leaves (32-126 µg/kg). In algae (chlorella vulgaris), about 3.5 µg/mg were detected (Borneff et al., 1968).

3. Biological Data Relevant to the Evaluation of Carcinogenic Risk to Man

3.1 Carcinogenicity and related studies in animals

(a) Skin application

Mouse: Three groups of 20 Swiss mice were painted thrice weekly with a 0.5, 0.1 or 0.01% solution of B(b)F in acetone. The highest dose produced papilloma in 100% and carcinomas in 90% of the animals within eight months; the intermediate dose produced papillomas in 65% and carcinomas in 85% within 12 months. At the lowest dose only one animal out of 10 survivors developed a papilloma after 14 months. No control group was run at the same time. In a parallel experiment with benzo(a)pyrene, repeated paintings of a 0.001% solution in acetone were effective (Wynder & Hoffmann, 1959b).

In a later experiment, a single painting of 1 mg in acetone produced no tumours among 20 Swiss mice in a study lasting 63 weeks. The same procedure followed by repeated paintings with croton resin produced papillomas in 18 and carcinomas in five of 20 mice (Van Duuren et al., 1966).

(b) Subcutaneous and/or intramuscular administration

Mouse: Among 16 male and 14 female mice of strain XVII nc/z given three s.c. injections of 0.6 mg B(b)F over a period of two months, 24 survived and 18 of these developed a sarcoma at the injection site with an average latent period of four-and-a-half months (Lacassagne et al., 1963).

3.2 Other relevant biological data

No data were available to the Working Group.

3.3 Observations in man

No data were available to the Working Group.

4. Comments on Data Reported and Evaluation

4.1 Animal data

B(b)F has produced skin tumours in mice following repeated skin paintings. The lowest carcinogenic dose for the mouse skin was at least ten times higher than that of benzo(a)pyrene. B(b)F is also an initiator of skin carcinogenesis in mice and produces local sarcomas after s.c. injections. It has not been tested by other routes in the mouse or in other species.

4.2 Human data

No case reports or epidemiological studies on the significance of B(b)F exposure to man are available. However, coal-tar and other materials which are known to be carcinogenic to man may contain B(b)F. The substance has also been detected in other environmental situations. The possible contribution of polycyclic aromatic hydrocarbons from some environmental sources to the overall carcinogenic risk to man is discussed in the preamble.

5. References

API Research Project 44 (1961) Selected Infrared Spectral Data, Vol. VI, No. 2312

Ayres, C.I. & Thornton, R.E. (1965) Determination of benzo(a)pyrene and related compounds in cigarette smoke. Beitr. Tabakforsch., 3, 285

Badger, G.M., Donnelly, J.K. & Spotswood, T.M. (1964) The formation of aromatic hydrocarbons at high temperatures. XIII. The pyrolysis of anthracene. Aust. J. Chem., 17, 1147

Badger, G.M., Donnelly, J.K. & Spotswood, T.M. (1965) The formation of aromatic hydrocarbons at high temperatures. XXIV. The pyrolysis of some tobacco constituents. Aust. J. Chem., 18, 1249

Bartle, K.D., Jones, D.W. & Matthews, R.S. (1969) High-field nuclear magnetic resonance spectra of some carcinogenic polynuclear hydrocarbons. Spectrochim. Acta, 25A, 1603

Beilsteins Handbuch der Organischen Chemie, 5, III, 2516

Borneff, J. & Fábián, B. (1966) Kanzerogene Substanzen in Speisefett und -öl. Arch. Hyg. (Muenchen), 150, 485

Borneff, J. & Fischer, R. (1962) Kanzerogene Substanzen in Wasser und Boden. XI. Polyzyklische, aromatische Kohlenwasserstoffe in Walderde. Arch. Hyg. (Muenchen), 146, 430

Borneff, J. & Fischer, R. (1963) Kanzerogene Substanzen in Wasser und Boden. XII. Polyzyklische, aromatische Kohlenwasserstoffe in Oberflächenwasser. Arch. Hyg. (Muenchen), 146, 572

Borneff, J. & Kunte, H. (1963) Kanzerogene Substanzen in Wasser und Boden. XIV. Weitere Untersuchungen über polyzyklische, aromatische Kohlenwasserstoffe in Erdproben. Arch. Hyg. (Muenchen), 147, 401

Borneff, J. & Kunte, H. (1964) Kanzerogene Substanzen in Wasser und Boden. XVI. Nachweis von polyzyklischen Aromaten in Wasserproben durch direkte Extraktion. Arch. Hyg. (Muenchen), 148, 585

Borneff, J. & Kunte, H. (1965) Kanzerogene Substanzen in Wasser und Boden. XVII. Über die Herkunft und Bewertung der polyzyklischen, aromatischen Kohlenwasserstoffe im Wasser. Arch. Hyg. (Muenchen), 149, 226

Borneff, J. & Kunte, H. (1967) Kanzerogene Substanzen in Wasser und Boden. XIX. Wirkung der Abwasserreinigung auf polyzyklische Aromaten. Arch. Hyg. (Muenchen), 151, 202

Borneff, J. & Kunte, H. (1969) Kanzerogene Substanzen in Wasser und Boden. XXVI. Routinemethode zur Bestimmung von polyzyklischen Aromaten im Wasser. Arch. Hyg. (Muenchen), 153, 220

Borneff, J., Selenka, F., Kunte, H. & Maximos, A. (1968) Experimental studies on the formation of polycyclic aromatic hydrocarbons in plants. Environ. Res., 2, 22

Bosco, G., Barsini, G. & Grella, A. (1967) Nuove indagini sulla presenza di idrocarburi policiclici aromatici nel pulviscolo atmosferico del centro storico della citta di Siena. Arch. environ. Hlth, 14, 285

Brocco, D., Cantuti, V. & Cartoni, G.P. (1970) Determination of polynuclear hydrocarbons in atmospheric dust by a combination of thin-layer and gas chromatography. J. Chromat., 49, 66

Chakraborty, B.B. & Long, R. (1967) Gas chromatographic analysis of polycyclic aromatic hydrocarbons in soot samples. Environ. Sci. Technol., 1, 828

Clar, E. (1964) Polycyclic Hydrocarbons, Vol. 2, London, New York, Academic Press; Berlin, Göttingen, Heidelberg, Springer-Verlag, p. 309

Cleary, G.J. (1963) Measurement of polycyclic aromatic hydrocarbons in the air of Sydney using very long alumina columns for separation. Int. J. air wat. Pollut., 7, 753

Colucci, J.M. & Begeman, C.R. (1965) The automotive contribution to air-borne polynuclear aromatic hydrocarbons in Detroit. J. air Pollut. Control Ass., 15, 113

Davis, H.J. (1969) Gas-chromatographic display of the polycyclic aromatic hydrocarbon fraction of cigarette smoke. Talanta, 16, 621

Del Vecchio, V., **Valori, P.**, Melchiorri, C. & Grella, A. (1970) Polycyclic aromatic hydrocarbons from gasoline-engine and liquefied petroleum gas engine exhausts. Pure appl. Chem., 24, 739

Edstrom, T. & Petro, B.A. (1968) Gel permeation chromatographic studies of polynuclear aromatic hydrocarbon materials. J. polymer Sci. C, 21, 171

Fábián, B. (1968a) Kanzerogene Substanzen in Speisefett und -öl. IV. Untersuchungen an Margarine, Pflanzenfett und Butter. Arch. Hyg. (Muenchen), 152, 231

Fábián, B. (1968b) Kanzerogene Substanzen in Speisefett und -öl. V. Untersuchungen an verschieden zubereiteten Bratwürsten. Arch. Hyg. (Muenchen), 152, 251

Fábián, B. (1969) Kanzerogene Substanzen in Speisefett und -öl. VI. Weitere Untersuchungen an Margarine und Schokolade. Arch. Hyg. (Muenchen), 153, 21

Fischer, R. (1970) Spektrophotometrisches Verfahren zur raschen Beurteilung von Russen auf ihren Gehalt an polycyclischen, aromatischen Kohlenwasserstoffen. Z. analyt. Chem., 249, 110

Fritz, W. (1968a) Zur Bildung canzerogener Kohlenwasserstoffe bei der thermischen Behandlung von Lebensmitteln. II. Das Rösten von Bohnenkaffee und Kaffee-Ersatzstoffen. Nahrung, 12, 799

Fritz, W. (1968b) Zur Bildung canzerogener Kohlenwasserstoffe bei der thermischen Behandlung von Lebensmitteln. IV. Der Einfluss des Frittierens. Nahrung, 12, 809

Fritz, W. (1969) Zur Lösungsverhalten der Polyaromaten beim Kochen von Kaffee-Ersatzstoffen und Bohnenkaffee. Dtsch. Lebensmitt.-Rdsch., 65, 83

Fryčka, J. (1972) Separation of polynuclear aromatic hydrocarbons by gas-solid chromatography on graphitized carbon black deposited on chromosorb W. J. Chromat., 65, 432

Gräf, W. & Diehl, W. (1966) Über den naturbedingten Normalpegel kanzerogener polyzyklischer Aromaten und seine Ursache. Arch. Hyg. (Muenchen), 150, 49

Hoffmann, D. & Wynder, E.L. (1962a) Analytical and biological studies on gasoline engine exhaust. Nat. Cancer Inst. Monogr., 9, 91

Hoffmann, D. & Wynder, E.L. (1962b) A study of air pollution carcinogenesis. II. The isolation and identification of polynuclear aromatic hydrocarbons from gasoline engine exhaust condensate. Cancer, 15, 93

Howard, J.W. & Teague, R.T. (1965) Extraction and estimation of polycyclic aromatic hydrocarbons added to milk. J. Ass. off. analyt. Chem., 48, 315

Kiryu, S. & Kuratsune, M. (1966) Polycyclic aromatic hydrocarbons in the cigarette tar produced by human smoking. Gann, 57, 317

Kruber, O. & Oberkobusch, R. (1952) Über neue Bestandteile des Steinkohlenteer-Pechs. Ber. dtsch. chem. Ges., 85 433

Lacassagne, A., Buu-Hoï, N.P., Zajdela, F., Lavit-Lamy, D. & Chalvet, O. (1963) Activité cancerogène d'hydrocarbures aromatiques polycycliques à noyau fluoranthène. Un. int. Cancr. Acta, 19, 490

Lyons, M.J. (1959) Vehicular exhausts. Identification of further carcinogens of the polycyclic aromatic hydrocarbon class. Brit. J. Cancer, 13, 126

Mallion, R.B. (1970) π-Electron ring currents in fluoranthene and related molecules. J. molec. Spectrosc., 35, 491

Masuda, Y. & Kuratsune, M. (1971) Polycyclic aromatic hydrocarbons in smoked fish, "katsuobushi". Gann, 62, 27

Masuda, Y., Mori, K. & Kuratsune, M. (1966a) Polycyclic aromatic hydrocarbons in common Japanese foods. I. Broiled fish, roasted barley, shoyu, and caramel. Gann, 57, 133

Masuda, Y., Mori, K., Hirohata, T. & Kuratsune, M. (1966b) Carcinogenesis in the esophagus. III. Polycyclic aromatic hydrocarbons and phenols in whisky. Gann, 57, 549

Masuda, Y., Mori, K. & Kuratsune, M. (1967) Polycyclic aromatic hydrocarbons formed by pyrolysis of carbohydrates, amino acids and fatty acids. Gann, 58, 69

Matsushita, H. & Suzuki, Y. (1969) Two-dimensional dual-band thin-layer chromatographic separation of polynuclear hydrocarbons. Bull. Chem. Soc. Japan, 42, 460

Matsushita, H., Esumi, Y. & Yamada, K. (1970) Identification of polynuclear hydrocarbons in air pollutants. Bunseki Kagaku, 19, 951

Savino, A. (1968) Determinazione per via gas chromatografica degli idrocarburi aromatici policiclici. Riv. ital. Igiene, 28, 56

Sawicki, E. (1964) The separation and analysis of polynuclear aromatic hydrocarbons present in the human environment. I-III. Chemist-Analyst, 53, 24, 56, 88

Sawicki, E. (1969) Fluorescence analysis in air pollution research. Talanta, 16, 1231

Sawicki, E., Hauser, T.R. & Stanley, T.W. (1960) Ultraviolet, visible and fluorescence spectral analysis of polynuclear hydrocarbons. Int. J. air Pollut., 2, 253

Scassellati-Sforzolini, G., Pascasio, F., Mastrandrea, F. & Savino, A. (1967) Attività cancerigena del fumo di sigaretta. Quantificazione degli idrocarburi aromatici policiclici presenti nella porzione aspirata. Riv. ital. Igiene, 27, 175

Schaad, R. (1970) Chromatographie (karzinogener) polyzyclische aromatischer Kohlenwasserstoffe. Chromat. Rev., 13, 61

Short, G.D. & Young, R. (1969) Charge-transfer chromatography of polycyclic hydrocarbons. Analyst, 94, 259

Strömberg, L.E. & Widmark, G. (1970) Qualitative determination of polyaromatic hydrocarbons in the air near gas-works retorts. J. Chromat., 47, 27

Titz, M. & Hochmann, P. (1967) Tables of quantum chemical data. XII. Energy characteristics of some benzo derivatives of acenaphthylene, fluoranthene and azulene. Coll. Cs. chem. Commun., 32, 2343

Tóth, L. (1971) Polyzyklische Kohlenwasserstoffe in geräuchertem Schinken und Bauchspeck. Fleischwirtschaft, 7, 1069

Van Duuren, B.L., Sivak, A., Segal, A., Orris, L. & Langseth, L. (1966) The tumor-producing agents of tobacco leaf and tobacco smoke condensate. J. nat. Cancer Inst., 37, 519

Wynder, E.L. & Hoffmann, D. (1959a) A study of tobacco carcinogenesis. VII. The role of higher polycyclic hydrocarbons. Cancer, 12, 1079

Wynder, E.L. & Hoffmann, D. (1959b) The carcinogenicity of benzofluoranthenes. Cancer, 12, 1194

Wynder, E.L. & Hoffmann, D. (1963) Ein experimenteller Beitrag zur Tabakrauchkanzerogenese. Dtsch. med. Wschr., 88, 623

BENZO(j)FLUORANTHENE*

1. Chemical and Physical Data

1.1 Synonyms

Chem. Abstr. No.: 205-82-3

7,8-Benzofluoranthene; 10,11-Benzofluoranthene; B(j)F

1.2 Chemical formula and molecular weight

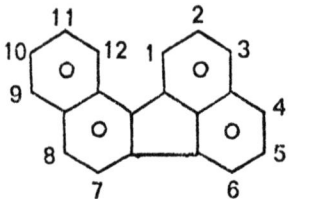

$C_{20}H_{12}$ Mol. wt: 252.32

1.3 Chemical and physical properties of the pure substance

(a) **Description**: Yellow plates or needles from alcohol. General description in Beilsteins handbook, and in Clar (1964).

(b) **Melting-point**: 165°C, 166-166.4°C

(c) **Absorption spectroscopy**: The ultra-violet absorption spectrum of benzo(j)fluoranthene (B(j)F) is described by Clar (1964), in ethanol; by Lang et al. (1957), in dioxane; and by Badger et al. (1965).

---

*Considered by the Working Group in Lyon, December 1972.

(d) <u>Identity and purity test</u>: B(j)F forms a picrate with a melting-point of 194-195°C (red needles); a complex with trinitrobenzene; orange needles from benzene and alcohol with a melting-point of 220-220.5°C; and a complex with 2,4,7-trinitro-fluorenone (orange-red, melting-point 255-256°C).

(e) <u>Solubility and/or volatility</u>: The substance is soluble in H_2SO_4 on heating. The solution has an olive-green colour. Distribution coefficients in the 4:1 cyclohexane/methanol-water system and in nitromethane/cyclohexane are indicated by Hoffmann & Wynder (1962a) as 14.8 and 1.75. Demisch & Wright (1963) have determined the coefficient as 10.2 for the hexane-aqueous monoethanolammonium/desoxycholate system.

(f) <u>Chemical reactivity</u>: Titz & Hochmann (1967) presented data on π-electron energy.

2. <u>Use and Occurrence</u>

(a) Analytical methods

For the separation of B(j)F from other substances by chromatography and subsequent spectroscopy, several procedures have been published. They include paper chromatography; column chromatography (Fischer, 1968); thin-layer chromatography (Fischer, 1968), used for detection in air (Strömberg & Widmark, 1970); fluorescence spectroscopy; and ultraviolet absorption spectroscopy (Strömberg & Widmark, 1970) and mass-spectroscopy (Strömberg & Widmark, 1970). References to analytical methods used for detection in various other media such as water, food, etc. can be found in the section on "Occurrence".

(<u>b</u>) Occurrence

<u>Exhaust</u>: Hoffmann & Wynder (1962a,b) isolated 17 mg/kg of exhaust tar from first-run gasoline engine exhaust, and 1.2 µg/minute run from automobile exhaust.

<u>Air</u>: Concentrations ranging from 62-205 mg/kg B(j)F were found in tar samples in the Detroit area (Colucci & Begeman, 1965); and in road dust 6-97 mg/kg, and in dust from air 0.62 mg/kg were found (Borneff & Kunte, 1965).

<u>Cigarette smoke</u>: In the smoke condensate of 100 cigarettes, Wynder & Hoffmann (1963) found 0.6 µg B(j)F, while Ayres & Thornton (1965) isolated approximately 3.7 µg B(j)F and benzo(b)fluoranthene[1]. In addition Wynder & Hoffmann (1959a) found 0.15-0.2 mg/kg in smoke condensate.

<u>Pyrolysis</u>: B(j)F is formed by pyrolysis of naphthalene at 750-770°C (Lang et al., 1957), of anthracene at 700-850°C (Badger et al., 1964), of the tobacco constituents dotriacontane and stigmasterol at 700°C, and of carbohydrates, amino acids and fatty acids at 700°C (400-3200 µg/kg), but not at 500°C (Masuda et al., 1967).

<u>Occupational exposure</u>: Fischer (1970) isolated an average of 7.3 mg/kg from soot samples, and Stefanescu & Stanescu (1968) found 300-3000 mg/1000 m^3 in different kinds of soot. B(j)F occurs in coal-tar (Kruber et al., 1953) at concentrations ranging from 450-630 mg/kg (Lijinsky et al., 1963); and in creosote oil 290 mg/kg have been found (Lijinsky et al., 1963).

---

[1] The two substances could not be completely separated.

Soil and water: In woodland soil samples of different areas in Germany concentrations of B(j)F and benzo(b)fluoranthene[1] ranged from 15-110 µg/kg (Borneff & Fischer, 1962; Borneff & Kunte, 1963). In the muddy deposits and in suspended matter of the Rhine river 1.8 and 1.3 mg/kg B(j)F and benzo(b)fluoranthene[1] were found (Borneff & Fischer, 1963). In drinking-water, concentrations ranged from 1.0-14.0 µg/m^3 B(j)F (Borneff & Kunte, 1964, 1969). In river and lake water a wide range of concentrations (53-17 840 µg/m^3) has been found, depending on the kind of water tested (whether or not it contained industrial effluents or bituminous contamination); while in surface water 4.6-150 µg/m^3 have been found, (Borneff & Kunte, 1964). As much as 29.6 mg/m^3 have been found in sewage water from household, industry and roads (Borneff & Kunte, 1967).

Food: In gas-broiled fish traces of up to 0.5 µg/kg B(j)F could be found (Masuda et al., 1966), while smoked or dried fish (wood smoke) could contain as much as 23 µg/kg (Masuda & Kuratsune, 1971). In the smoke of gas- and electric-broiled fish B(j)F was also detected (Masuda et al., 1966).

Fresh sausages contained 0.18 µg/kg, and, when grilled or fried, up to 15 µg/kg (Fábián, 1968b). In olive oil, plant cooking fat, plant oil and coconut oil, concentrations ranged from 0.8-4.4 µg/kg (Borneff & Fábián, 1966; Fábián, 1968a), and in margarine from 2.3-10.5 µg/kg (Fábián, 1968a), the concentration being reduced by treatment with activated charcoal and steam (Fábián, 1969). In fat, the concentration could be

---

[1] The two substances could not be completely separated.

reduced by controlled laboratory heating (Borneff & Fábián, 1966).

3. Biological Data Relevant to the Evaluation of Carcinogenic Risk to Man

3.1 Carcinogenicity and related studies in animals

(a) Skin application

Mouse: Thrice weekly skin paintings of groups of 30 Swiss mice with a 0.1 or 0.5% solution of B(j)F in acetone induced carcinomas within seven to nine months in at least 95% of the animals, as well as producing papillomas (Wynder & Hoffmann, 1959b).

3.2 Other relevant biological data

None were available to the Working Group.

3.3 Observations in man

None were available to the Working Group.

4. Comments on Data Reported and Evaluation

4.1 Animal data

B(j)F has only been tested in mice by repeated skin painting, when a high incidence of skin carcinomas was obtained. It has not been tested by other routes in the mouse or in other species.

4.2 Human data

No case reports or epidemiological studies on the significance of B(j)F exposure to man are available. However, coal-tar and other materials which are known to be carcinogenic to man may contain B(j)F. The substance has also been detected in other environmental situations. The possible contribution of polycyclic aromatic hydrocarbons from some environmental sources to the overall carcinogenic risk to man is discussed in the preamble.

5. References

Ayres, C.I. & Thornton, R.E. (1965) Determination of benzo(a)-pyrene and related compounds in cigarette smoke. Beitr. Tabakforsch., 3, 285

Badger, G.M., Donnelly, J.K. & Spotswood, T.M. (1964) The formation of aromatic hydrocarbons at high temperatures. XIII. The pyrolysis of anthracene. Aust. J. Chem., 17 1147

Badger, G.M., Donnelly, J.K. & Spotswood, T.M. (1965) The formation of aromatic hydrocarbons at high temperatures. XXIV. The pyrolysis of some tobacco constituents. Aust. J. Chem., 18, 1249

Beilsteins Handbuch der Organischen Chemie, 5, III, 2515

Borneff, J. & Fábián, B. (1966) Kanzerogene Substanzen in Speisefett und -öl. Arch. Hyg. (Muenchen), 150, 485

Borneff, J. & Fischer, R. (1962) Kanzerogene Substanzen in Wasser und Boden. XI. Polyzyklische, aromatische Kohlenwasserstoffe in Walderde. Arch. Hyg. (Muenchen), 146, 430

Borneff, J. & Fischer, R. (1963) Kanzerogene Substanzen in Wasser und Boden. XI. Polyzyklische, aromatische Kohlenwasserstoffe in Oberflächenwasser. Arch. Hyg. (Muenchen), 146, 572

Borneff, J. & Kunte, H. (1963) Kanzerogene Substanzen in Wasser und Boden. XIV. Weitere Untersuchungen über polyzyklische, aromatische Kohlenwasserstoffe in Erdproben. Arch. Hyg. (Muenchen), 147, 401

Borneff, J. & Kunte, H. (1964) Kanzerogene Substanzen in Wasser und Boden. XVI. Nachweis von polyzyklischen Aromaten in Wasserproben durch direkte Extraktion. Arch. Hyg. (Muenchen), 148, 585

Borneff, J. & Kunte, H. (1965) Kanzerogene Substanzen in Wasser und Boden. XVII. Über die Herkunft und Bewertung der polyzyklischen, aromatischen Kohlenwasserstoffe im Wasser. Arch. Hyg. (Muenchen), 149, 226

Borneff, J. & Kunte, H. (1967) Kanzerogene Substanzen in Wasser und Boden. XIX. Wirkung der Abwasserreinigung auf polyzyklische Aromaten. Arch. Hyg. (Muenchen), 151, 202

Borneff, J. & Kunte, H. (1969) Kanzerogene Substanzen in Wasser und Boden. XXVI. Routinemethode zur Bestimmung von polyzyklischen Aromaten in Wasser. Arch. Hyg. (Muenchen), 153, 220

Clar, E. (1964) Polycyclic Hydrocarbons, Vol. 2, London, New York, Academic Press; Berlin, Göttingen, Heidelberg, Springer-Verlag, pp. 312, 314

Colucci, J.M. & Begeman, C.R. (1965) The automotive contribution to air-borne polynuclear aromatic hydrocarbons in Detroit. J. air Pollut. Control Ass., 15, 113

Demisch, R.R. & Wright, G.F. (1963) The distribution of polynuclear aromatic hydrocarbons between aqueous and nonaqueous phases. Canad. J. Biochem., 41, 1655

Fábián, B. (1968a) Kanzerogene Substanzen in Speisefett und -öl. IV. Untersuchungen an Margarine, Pflanzenfett und Butter. Arch. Hyg. (Muenchen), 152, 231

Fábián, B. (1968b) Kanzerogene Substanzen in Speisefett und -öl. V. Untersuchungen an verschieden zubereiteten Bratwürsten. Arch. Hyg. (Muenchen), 152, 251

Fábián, B. (1969) Kanzerogene Substanzen in Speisefett und -öl. VI. Weitere Untersuchungen an Margarine und Schokolade. Arch. Hyg. (Muenchen), 153, 21

Fischer, R. (1968) Production of benzo(j)fluoranthene for comparison purposes in chromatography. Chromatographia, 1, 403

Fischer, R. (1970) Spektrophotometrisches Verfahren zur raschen Beurteilung von Russen auf ihren Gehalt an polycyclischen, aromatischen Kohlenwasserstoffen. Z. analyt. Chem., 249, 110

Hoffmann, D. & Wynder, E.L. (1962a) Analytical and biological studies on gasoline engine exhaust. Nat. Cancer Inst. Monogr., 9, 91

Hoffmann, D. & Wynder, E.L. (1962b) A study of air pollution carcinogenesis. II. The isolation and identification of polynuclear aromatic hydrocarbons from gasoline engine exhaust condensate. Cancer, 15, 93

Kruber, O., Oberkobusch, R. & Rappen, L. (1953) Über das 10,11- und 11,12-Benzofluoranthen im Steinkohlenteer-Pech. Ber. dtsch. chem. Ges., 86, 534

Lang, K.F., Buffleb, H. & Kalowy, J. (1957) Die Pyrolyse des Naphthalins. Chem. Ber., 90, 2888

Lijinsky, W., Domsky, I., Mason, G., Ramahi, H.Y. & Safavi, T. (1963) The chromatographic determination of trace amounts of polynuclear hydrocarbons in petrolatum, mineral oil and coal-tar. Analyt. Chem., 35, 952

Masuda, Y. & Kuratsune, M. (1971) Polycyclic aromatic hydrocarbons in smoked fish, "katsuobushi". Gann, 62, 27

Masuda, Y., Mori, K. & Kuratsune, M. (1966) Polycyclic aromatic hydrocarbons in common Japanese foods. I. Broiled fish, roasted barley, shoyu, and caramel. Gann, 57, 133

Masuda, Y., Mori, K. & Kuratsune, M. (1967) Polycyclic aromatic hydrocarbons formed by pyrolysis of carbohydrates, amino acids and fatty acids. Gann, 58, 69

Stefanescu, A. & Stanescu, L. (1968) Der Gefährdungsgrad unter Einwirkung der aromatischen polynuklearen Kohlenwasserstoffe beim Fabrikationsprozess von Russ. II. Die Gefährdung durch einige krebserzeugende Kohlenwasserstoffe und ihre Bestimmung in der Luft. Z. ges. Hyg., 14, 599

Strömberg, L.E. & Widmark, G. (1970) Qualitative determination of polyaromatic hydrocarbons in the air near gas-works retorts. J. Chromat., 47, 27

Titz, M. & Hochmann, P. (1967) Tables of quantum chemical data. XII. Energy characteristics of some benzo derivatives of acenaphthylene, fluoranthene and azulene. Coll. Cs. chem. Commun., 32, 2343

Wynder, E.L. & Hoffmann, D. (1959a) A study of tobacco carcinogenesis. VII. The role of higher polycyclic hydrocarbons. Cancer, 12, 1079

Wynder, E.L. & Hoffmann, D. (1959b) The carcinogenicity of benzofluoranthenes. Cancer, 12, 1194

Wynder, E.L. & Hoffmann, D. (1963) Ein experimenteller Beitrag zur Tabakrauchkanzerogenese. Dtsch. med. Wschr., 88, 623

BENZO(a)PYRENE*

1. Chemical and Physical Data

1.1 Synonyms

Chem. Abstr. No.: 50-32-8

3,4-Benzopyrene; 1,2-Benzopyrene; 3,4-Benzpyrene; 1,2-Benzpyrene; B(a)P

1.2 Chemical formula and molecular weight

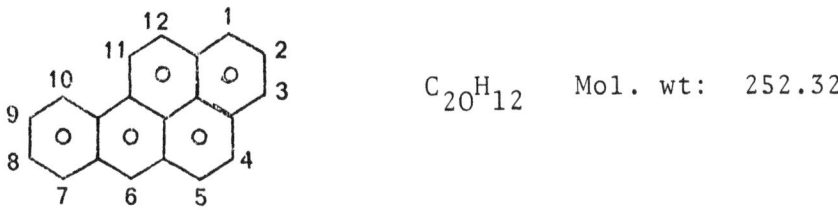

$C_{20}H_{12}$ Mol. wt: 252.32

1.3 Chemical and physical properties of the pure substance

(a) *Description*: Pale yellow needles or plates from benzene/methanol. Solutions in benzene show a blue or violet fluorescence. A solution in concentrated sulphuric acid is orange-red with a green fluorescence. General description in Beilsteins handbook and in Clar (1964).

(b) *Boiling-point*: 310-312°C/10 mm; 475°C/760 mm

(c) *Melting-point*: 176.5-177.5°C; 179-179.3°C

(d) *Density*: 1.351 (Kronberger & Weiss, 1944)

(e) *Absorption spectroscopy*: The ultra-violet absorption spectrum is described in Perkampus et al. (1967),

---

* Considered by the Working Group in Lyon, December 1972.

in heptane; by Clar (1964), Van Duuren (1958), Stanley et al. (1967), Howard et al. (1966a,b), Sawicki et al. (1960a,b), and Strömberg & Widmark (1970a), in ethanol. The fluorescence spectrum is described by Van Duuren (1958), Howard et al. (1966a,b); Reske & Stauff (1963), in water; and by Sawicki et al. (1960b), in sulphuric acid; and the low temperature luminescence characteristics are measured by Hood & Winefordner (1968). The infrared absorption spectrum is contained in the collection of spectra by Mecke & Langenbucher (1965) and Pouchert (1971); the mass spectrum was described by Strömberg & Widmark (1970a) and the nuclear magnetic resonance spectrum by Bartle et al. (1969) and Haigh et al. (1970).

(f) <u>Identity and purity test</u>: Benzo(a)pyrene (B(a)P) forms a picrate (dark red needles from benzene, melting-point 197-198°C) and a red complex with 1,3,5-trinitrobenzene (melting-point 227-228.5°C from benzene).

(g) <u>Solubility and/or volatility</u>: A solubility of 0.004 mg/l of water at 27°C was found by Davis et al. (1942) and 0.012 mg/l by Wilk & Schwab (1968). B(a)P is soluble in benzene, toluene and xylene and sparingly soluble in ethanol and methanol. Solubility in aqueous caffein is higher than in water (Eisenbrand & Baumann, 1970); also, native DNA has a solubilizing effect (Boyland & Green, 1962a,b). The distribution coefficient in the nitromethane/cyclohexane system was determined as 1.81 by Müller et al. (1967) and as 2.05 by Grimmer (1961).

(h) <u>Stability</u>: B(a)P oxidizes in benzene under the influence of light and air (Allsop, 1940; Boyland, 1933).

(i) <u>Chemical reactivity</u>: Hydrogenation with platinum oxide gives 4,5-dihydrobenzo(a)pyrene, 7,8,9,10-tetrahydrobenzo(a)pyrene and perhydrobenzo(a)pyrene (Lijinsky & Zechmeister, 1953). On oxidation with chromic acid or ozone, B(a)P yields benzo(a)pyrene-1,6-quinone and benzo(a)pyrene-3,6-quinone, and on further oxidation benzanthrone dicarboxylic anhydride (Vollmann et al., 1937; Moriconi et al., 1961). Electrophilic substitution occurs mainly in position 6.

2. Use and Occurrence

(a) Analytical methods

Several chromatographic procedures for the separation of B(a)P from other substances and for its spectroscopic determination have been published and are extensively reviewed by Sawicki (1964) and by Schaad (1970). They include paper chromatography (Siddiqui & Wagner, 1972); column chromatography, used for detection in water (Siddiqui & Wagner, 1972); thin-layer chromatography (Siddiqui & Wagner, 1972), used for detection in air (Sawicki et al., 1970a,b,c; Strömberg & Widmark, 1970b); gas chromatography (Bhatia, 1971; Gouw et al., 1970; Fryčka, 1972), used for detection in air (Searl et al., 1970; Strömberg & Widmark, 1970b); high-speed liquid-liquid chromatography (Schmit et al., 1971); gel chromatography (Edstrom & Petro, 1968; Oelert, 1969), used for detection in exhaust (Gladen, 1972), for detection in air (Klimisch & Reese, 1972) and for detection in cigarette smoke (Stedman et al.,

1968); sublimation, used for detection in air (Monkman et al., 1970); ultra-violet absorption spectroscopy (Gladen, 1972; Searl et al., 1970; Siddiqui & Wagner, 1972; Strömberg & Widmark, 1970b); and fluorescence spectroscopy (Sawicki et al., 1970a,b,c; Monkman et al., 1970). References to analytical methods used for detection in various other media, such as air, water, food, etc., can be found in the section on "Occurrence".

(<u>b</u>) <u>Occurrence</u>

<u>Exhaust</u>: The amounts of B(a)P present in the exhaust of internal combustion engines were determined with a variety of workloads and fuels and with reference to a number of differing parameters. Automobile engines using gasoline as fuel produced 330 mg/kg of soot under idling conditions (zero load) (Falk et al., 1958), while the average of five sampling periods of normal run exhaust soot amounted to 220 mg/kg of particulate matter (Sawicki et al., 1962b). From a gasoline engine operated on a simulated city driving schedule 31.5 mg/kg of exhaust tar were isolated (Hoffmann & Wynder, 1962a), and 2.2-9.6 µg/minute run were found (Hoffmann & Wynder, 1962b, 1963). On a simulated working schedule with a 1000 kg load, 20 mg/1000 m^3 of exhaust were found (Del Vecchio et al., 1970). The output of eight automobiles was 2.9-33.5 µg/mile (Hangebrauck et al., 1966).

Engines using diesel fuel on full load produced some 12 mg/kg of soot (Falk et al., 1958), while under various combustions two-cycle engines produced 0.1-3.1 mg/1000 m^3 of exhaust and four-cycle engines 0.6-7.4 mg/1000 m^3 (Reckner et al., 1965). The output of four trucks was about 40 µg/mile (Hangebrauck et al., 1966).

Engines using liquified petroleum gas produced 10.9 mg/1000 m^3 at full working load and 3.8 mg/1000 m^3 under idling conditions (zero load) (Del Vecchio et al., 1970). The contribution of automobiles to levels of atmospheric B(a)P varied between 5-42%; this percentage being influenced by seasonal factors (Sawicki, 1967).

Air: The concentration of B(a)P in the atmosphere has been reviewed repeatedly (Sawicki, 1967; Kotin & Falk, 1963). Concentrations depend on the geographic location, the presence of nearby sources of pollution such as traffic highways or industries, and on the season. In general, concentrations were greater in urban than in non-urban areas (up to 100 times more in urban areas) and greater in winter than in summer (up to 100 times) and during periods of increased smoke in the atmosphere.

Detailed studies of air pollution in a variety of cities in Europe (Bosco et al., 1967; Commins & Waller, 1967; Grimmer, 1966; Stocks et al., 1961), USA (Colucci & Begeman, 1965; Conlee et al., 1967; DeMaio & Corn, 1966; Epstein et al., 1966; Sawicki et al., 1962b, 1965a,b; Von Lehmden et al., 1965), Australia (Cleary, 1963; Cleary & Sullivan, 1965) and South Africa (Louw, 1965) have been reported. Seasonal variations were recorded; thus, winter values ranged from 0.6-104 µg/1000 m^3, and summer values from 0.03-4 µg/1000 m^3 (Bosco et al., 1967; Colucci & Begeman, 1965; DeMaio & Corn, 1966; Sawicki et al., 1962b; Von Lehmden et al., 1965; Waller & Commins, 1967).

In London, during a period in which smoke condensation was high (December 1957), a concentration as high as 2220 µg/1000 m^3 was recorded (Commins & Waller, 1967), but after that winter values did not exceed 54 µg/1000 m^3. In Sydney, samples from four different areas of the town showed concentrations ranging from 2.5-6.5 µg/1000 m^3 (Cleary, 1963), and in three South African cities 16-146 µg/1000 m^3 have been found (Louw, 1965).

In industrial areas B(a)P was found in concentrations of 30-50 mg/kg (Dikun & Nikberg, 1958), and the air in an old industrial town (Irkutsk) contained considerably more B(a)P than did that of a new industrial town (Angarsk) (Grushko et al., 1958).

Examination of particulates or extracts in six US cities gave the following results: 80-800 µg/g of benzene soluble fraction (Sawicki et al., 1965a), and 110-670 µg/g of organic atmospheric particulate matter (Epstein et al., 1966).

Cigarette smoke: B(a)P has been reported in a great number of studies from all over the world to be present in cigarette smoke in amounts ranging from 0.2-12.2 µg/100 cigarettes (Surgeon General's Report, 1964; Wynder & Hoffmann, 1967). The average of 10 values selected on the basis of adequacy of the analytical procedure was in the order of 1.6 µg/100 cigarettes; however a loss of B(a)P during the process of fractionation and purification is likely to occur (Surgeon General's Report, 1964). Elmenhorst & Grimmer (1968) detected an average concentration of 1.31 mg/kg in cigarette smoke condensate.

Pyrolysis: B(a)P has been produced by pyrolysis of anthracene at 950°C (16 000 mg/kg) (Badger et al., 1964), of dicetyl at 800°C (370 mg/kg) (Lam, 1956a), of carbohydrates, amino acids and fatty acids at 700°C

(1.2-88.8 mg/kg) and at 500°C (up to 0.14 mg/kg) (Masuda et al., 1967) and of different tobacco constituents at 650°C (cured tobacco, up to 0.8 mg/kg) (Gilbert & Lindsey, 1957), at 700°C (dotriacontane, 1300 mg/kg; stigmasterol, 6000 mg/kg; aliphatic hydrocarbons, 30 mg/kg) (Badger et al., 1965; Lam, 1956b) and at 800°C (aliphatic hydrocarbons, 340 mg/kg) (Lam, 1956b). The amount of B(a)P found among the pyrolysis products of various materials, including agar-agar, natural dyes, humectants, glues, starches and logwood, varied between 6 µg/kg of starting material for extract of logwood and 470 µg/kg for agar-agar (Kroeller, 1965a,b).

Occupational exposure: The isolation of B(a)P from coal-tar dates back to 1933 (Cook et al., 1933). Kreyberg (1959) isolated B(a)P concentrations ranging from 180-7300 µg/1000 m^3 from the air of two gas works and one electrical plant. In gas works retort houses mean concentrations ranging from 1.4-4.8 mg/1000m^3 and maximum concentrations of 2300 mg/1000 m^3 have been measured (Lawther et al., 1965). Sawicki et al. (1965b) found 0.4 mg/1000 m^3 in air polluted by coal-tar pitch fumes, up to 2700 mg/1000 m^3 in industrial effluents and 1000 mg/1000 m^3 in domestic coal combustion stack effluents. In the workers' atmosphere in coal and pitch coking plants average concentrations ranging from 0.3-35 mg/1000 m^3 (Masek, 1971) have been found. B(a)P is present in all kinds of soot and smoke. Hamm & Toth (1970) detected it in tar and smoke from smoke houses, and Rhee & Bratzler (1968) in wood smoke. In carbon black soot, 20-40 mg/kg have been found (Falk et al., 1958), and in different kinds of soot 52-510 mg/1000 m^3 (Stefanescu & Stanescu, 1968) and 5.3 mg/kg (Fischer, 1970) have been detected.

The emission levels of B(a)P from heat generation sources ranged from 19-400 000 µg/10^6 Btu[1] heat input (coal) and 20-200 µg/10^6 Btu heat input (gas). From incineration and open burning (of municipal refuse, automobile tyres, etc.) the emission levels ranged from 0.016-3.3 mg/kg of particulate matter for a municipal incinerator, 58-180 mg/kg of particulate matter for a commercial incinerator, and 11-1100 mg/kg of particulate matter in open burning (Hangebrauck et al., 1964).

Average values for five sampling periods at a downtown garage were 33 µg/1000 m^3 (Sawicki et al., 1962b), and air polluted by coal-tar fumes during a sidewalk tarring operation contained 78 mg/1000 m^3 (Sawicki et al., 1962a). Vapours produced at 300°C from melted coal-tar contained up to 44 g/kg and the solid tar 30 g/kg (Bonnet, 1962). From measurements at three different places close to a workman he calculated that the man would inhale 0.26-2.98 mg/hour depending on the temperature of the tar. Up to 12.5 g/kg were found in coal-tar and coal-tar pitch (Lijinsky et al., 1963; Sawicki et al., 1962b; Shabad et al., 1970; Wallcave et al., 1971). 0.1-27 mg/kg B(a)P were also detected in petroleum asphalt (Wallcave et al., 1971), 0.34 µg/kg in wood tar (Shabad et al., 1970), 0.3-1 µg/kg in bituminous coal (Tye et al., 1966), 0.14-0.2 µg/kg in creosote oil (Lijinsky et al., 1963), up to 0.1 µg/kg in shale oil (Berenblum & Schoental, 1943b), 23 µg/kg in the commercial solvent hexane (Lijinsky & Raha, 1961) and up to 0.55 µg/kg in asbestos (Harington, 1962).

---

[1] British thermal unit

Soil and water: For a review of B(a)P concentrations in soil see Shabad et al. (1971). Studies on the B(a)P content of soil have been carried out in many countries, and concentrations vary depending on the distance from a source of pollution. Air pollution is considered to be the main source; however, microorganisms in the soil may either metabolize or accumulate B(a)P (Shabad, 1968).

In non-industrial areas (forest, wood and sand samples in Germany, France, Bohemia and USA; and lava and humus soil in Iceland) concentrations ranging from 0 (Iceland) - 127 µg/kg have been found (Blumer, 1961; Borneff & Fischer, 1962; Borneff & Kunte, 1963; Fritz & Engst, 1971; Grimmer et al., 1972; Mallet & Héros, 1962; Zdrazil & Picha, 1966), and up to 1300 µg/kg were found by Blumer (1961) in forest samples. In studies concerning Paris, Moscow and a Bohemian town and their vicinities, concentrations ranging from 0-939 µg/kg have been found, depending on the degree of urbanization and the amount of traffic (Perdriau, 1963; Shabad, 1968; Zdrazil & Picha, 1966). B(a)P has been found in soil near traffic highways, up to 2000 µg/kg (Zdrazil & Picha, 1966), and in the soil of an oil refinery plant, 200 mg/kg (Shabad, 1968); and up to 650 mg/kg have been detected in soil polluted by coal-tar pitch (Fritz & Engst, 1971). B(a)P content was found to be higher in the region of an airfield than at control points and to be gradually reduced with increasing distance from the source of pollution (Smirnov, 1970); and in an airfield sample from Iceland 785 µg/kg have been found (Grimmer et al., 1972).

Andelman & Suess (1970) summarize B(a)P content in water. In drinking-water, 0.1-23.4 µg/m^3 B(a)P have been found (Borneff & Kunte, 1964, 1969). In surface water, concentrations ranged from 0.6-114 µg/m^3 (Borneff & Kunte, 1964), and in several samples of effluents a wide range of concentrations (1-1840 µg/m^3) has been found, possibly due to industrial effluents or to bituminous contamination (Borneff & Kunte, 1965). As much as 34.5 mg/m^3 were determined in sewage water from household, trade and industrial sources (Borneff & Kunte, 1967).

Food: In meat or fish the amount of B(a)P present depends on the method of cooking: time of exposure, distance from the heat source and whether or not the melted fat is allowed to drop into the heat source. In broiled meat or sausages 0.17-0.63 µg/kg were found (Grimmer & Hildebrandt, 1967a), and 0.9 µg/kg were detected in gas-broiled fish (Masuda et al., 1966b). In charcoal-broiled or barbecued meat concentrations ranged from 2.6-11.2 µg/kg (Lijinsky & Ross, 1967; Lijinsky & Shubik, 1964, 1965), and as much as 50.4 µg/kg were detected in one T-bone steak (long cooking time) (Lijinsky & Ross, 1967). In smoked fish, concentrations ranging from traces to 2.1 µg/kg have been found (Bailey & Dungal, 1958; Dungal, 1959; Gorelova et al., 1960; Grimmer & Hildebrandt, 1967a; Lijinsky & Shubik, 1965; Masuda & Kuratsune, 1971), and Masuda & Kuratsune (1971) found up to 37 µg/kg in Japanese smoked fish. In smoked meat, ham and sausages 0.02-14.6 µg/kg were found (Bailey & Dungal, 1958; Hamm & Toth, 1970; Malanoski et al., 1968; Toth, 1971), and Thorsteinsson (1969) detected up to 23 µg/kg in Icelandic home smoked meat and 107 µg/kg if the meat was hung close to the stove.

In fruit, vegetables and cereals the B(a)P content depends on their source (closeness to industrial areas or traffic highways). In fruit and vegetables, the following amounts of B(a)P were found: salad, 2.8-5.3 µg/kg; spinach, 7.4 µg/kg; tomatoes, 0.2 µg/kg; kale, 12.6-48.1 µg/kg; soya beans, 3.1 µg/kg; apples, 0.1-0.5 µg/kg; other fruits, 2-8 µg/kg. Washing of kale removed only 10% of the quantity (Fritz & Engst, 1971; Grimmer & Düvel, 1970; Grimmer & Hildebrandt, 1965a; Hettche, 1971). Cereals were contaminated to variable degrees (0.2-4.1 µg/kg) (Grimmer & Düvel, 1970; Grimmer & Hildebrandt, 1965b), and the amount present is transferred to flour and bread (Fritz, 1968c).

In different kinds of crude vegetable oils, concentrations ranging from 0.9-15 µg/kg were found, and up to 43.7 µg/kg were detected in crude coconut oil (Biernoth & Rost, 1967; Grimmer & Hildebrandt, 1967b). B(a)P has been detected in refined vegetable oils (Jung & Morand, 1963), and concentrations range from 0.4-36 µg/kg (Biernoth & Rost, 1968; Borneff & Fábián, 1966; Howard et al., 1966b). In coconut fat, up to 62 µg/kg have been detected (Biernoth & Rost, 1968), and 0.2-6.8 µg/kg have been found in margarine (Fábián, 1968, 1969; Fritz, 1968a). The B(a)P content of oils and fats decreased slightly with frying (Berner & Biernoth, 1969; Fritz, 1968d).

In roasted coffee, concentrations ranged from 0.1-4 µg/kg (Fritz, 1968b, 1969; Kuratsune & Hueper, 1960; Maier & Stender, 1969), while as much as 15 µg were found in heavily roasted malt coffee (Fritz, 1966, 1969).

In tea, concentrations ranged from 3.9-21.3 µg/kg (Grimmer & Hildebrandt, 1966). In baker's dry yeast, Grimmer & Wilhelm (1969) detected 1.8-40.4 µg/kg, while dietetic yeast or feed yeasts grown on mineral oil show a lower content. Masuda et al. (1966a) found 0.04 µg/kg in one of 15 brands of whisky; and in prunes dried by different methods, concentrations ranged from 0.2-1.5 µg/kg (Ruchkovskii et al., 1969).

Other material: B(a)P has been detected in algae (chlorella vulgaris) (Borneff et al., 1968) and in leaves from different kinds of trees (Gräf & Diehl, 1966; Mallet & Héros, 1962). In furnace blacks, automobile tyres and rubber stoppers concentrations have also been found, and these did not diminish on processing, aging or wear (Falk et al., 1951; Smith et al., 1968).

3. Biological Data Relevant to the Evaluation of Carcinogenic Risk to Man

3.1 Carcinogenicity and related studies in animals

(a) Oral administration

Mouse: B(a)P has been shown by several investigators and in different laboratories to produce benign and malignant tumours in the forestomach (Hartwell, 1951; Shubik & Hartwell, 1957, 1969; Thompson & Co., 1971; Tracor/Jitco, 1973a,b). A single intragastric administration of 0.2 mg/mouse in PEG produced a total of 14 tumours in five animals out of 11. Tumours appeared following single doses of 0.05 and 0.012 mg/mouse in 0/9 and 2/10 mice (Peirce, 1961).

The effects of feeding diets containing different concentrations of B(a)P to mice were investigated in a series of studies (Rigdon & Neal, 1966; Neal & Rigdon, 1967; Rigdon & Neal, 1969). An estimation of the effective schedule of treatment is impaired by the fact that not all groups were treated for the same period of time and that age at start ranged between 17 and 116 days. No stomach tumours were found at the end of a 110-day treatment with diets containing up to 30 ppm B(a)P. Tumour incidences lower than 10% were observed in mice receiving 40-45 ppm for 110 days, whereas mice bearing stomach tumours exceeded 70% among those given 50-250 ppm B(a)P for 122-197 days. A diet containing 250 ppm B(a)P fed for different periods of time produced the following incidences of tumours of the forestomach: one day of feeding, 0%; two to four days of feeding, 10%; five to seven days of feeding, 30-40%; 30 days of feeding, 100% (Neal & Rigdon, 1967). In a subsequent experiment, a diet containing 250 ppm B(a)P fed for 140 days to mice of the same strain starting at 18-30 days of age was reported to have produced leukaemias and lung adenomas in addition to stomach tumours (Rigdon & Neal, 1969). The ability of B(a)P to produce lung adenomas when administered in the diet was confirmed in another study (Wattenberg & Leong, 1970).

Rat: A single oral administration of 100 mg B(a)P to 50-day-old female Sprague Dawley rats produced mammary tumours in eight out of nine animals (Huggins & Yang, 1962). In another study with Sprague Dawley rats of both sexes aged three-and-a-half months at the beginning of the experiment, daily doses of 2.5 mg B(a)P/rat induced papillomas in the oesophagus and forestomach in three out of 40 animals (Gibel, 1964).

Hamster: Bi-weekly administration of 2-5 mg B(a)P in oil by stomach tube produced five papillomas of the stomach in 67 hamsters treated for one to five months, seven papillomas and two carcinomas in 18 treated for six to nine months and five papillomas in eight treated for 10-11 months (Dontenwill & Mohr, 1962). In a subsequent experiment with 13 hamsters, a diet containing 500 ppm B(a)P given for four days/week for up to 14 months caused a total of 12 tumours (two in the oesophagus, eight in the forestomach and two in the intestine) in eight hamsters (Chu & Malmgren, 1965).

(b) Skin application

Mouse: Many experiments with repeated applications of B(a)P have been performed since the original demonstration by Cook et al. (1933) and Cook (1933) that B(a)P induces skin tumours in mice. Some dose-response studies, including a no-effect dose level, have been reported, and these indicate that the threshold dose is affected by the strain of mouse and the solvent chosen. Thrice weekly applications of B(a)P in acetone to CAF1 mice induced no tumours at a concentration of 0.0005%, a total of six papillomas and two carcinomas among 19 mice at a concentration of 0.001% and increasing incidence of benign and malignant tumours with progressively shorter latent periods at higher doses. In Swiss and C57BL mice, tumours were not induced at concentrations of 0.001% or less, whereas incidences approaching 100% were found at 0.005% or higher concentrations (Wynder et al., 1957). In another study, toluene was used as the solvent and SWR, C3HeB and A/He mice were painted thrice weekly with different amounts of B(a)P. In SWR and C3HeB mice the lowest effective dose was 0.38 µg B(a)P per application, with an obvious dose-response relationship above this dose for both the percentage of tumour-bearing animals and the shortening of the latent period; doses of 0.15 µg were ineffective. On the other hand, in A/He mice, paintings with 0.15-3.8 µg B(a)P were ineffective, whereas tumours were induced following doses of 19 µg or more (Poel, 1963). With acetone as the solvent and using Swiss mice, borderline activity was detected following thrice weekly painting with 0.1-1 µg B(a)P, while tumours appeared with 3 µg and above (Roe et al., 1970).

The modifying effect of solvents on the carcinogenicity of B(a)P is well demonstrated by a comparison between the effects of thrice weekly paintings with different concentrations of B(a)P either in n-dodecane/decalin (50:50 mixture) or in decalin on C3H/He mice. When n-dodecane/decalin was the solvent, five malignant tumours appeared among 24 mice painted with the lowest concentration, i.e., 0.00002%, and the tumour incidence increased at higher doses. With decalin, no skin tumours developed in any of the mice below the 0.02% concentration (Bingham & Falk, 1969).

Following repeated paintings of 0.05% solutions in dioxane on HA/ICR/Mil Swiss albino mice, the time at which 50% of the mice had tumours was six months for B(a)P, nine months for dibenzo(a,h)pyrene, 11 months for dibenzo(a,i)pyrene and more than 15 months for dibenzo(a,e)pyrene (Hoffmann & Wynder, 1966). The activity of B(a)P is in the same order of magnitude as that of dibenzo(a,h)pyrene since in other experiments on Swiss mice repeated paintings with a 0.001% solution of B(a)P in acetone produced papillomas in 43% and carcinomas in 3% of the mice and the same concentration of dibenzo(a,h)pyrene produced papillomas in 30% and carcinomas in 30%. On the other hand, a 0.01% solution of either compound produced both papillomas and carcinomas in over 90% of the mice with similar latent periods (Wynder & Hoffmann, 1959).

Single applications of 752 µg B(a)P in toluene to 13 C57L mice caused papillomas in two animals and a carcinoma in one; a dose of 94 µg was ineffective (Poel, 1959).

B(a)P is an initiator of skin carcinogenesis: this has been confirmed repeatedly since the original observation of Salaman & Gwynn (1951).

Rat: The rat has been used in experiments to produce skin carcinogenesis to a much lesser extent than has the mouse. In an experiment lasting 150 days, Nakano (1937) produced seven papillomas and four carcinomas among 15 rats painted weekly with a 0.5-1% solution of B(a)P in benzene.

Hamster: Bi-weekly paintings with a 0.01% solution of B(a)P in acetone for 40 weeks did not produce skin tumours among 10 Syrian golden hamsters. A total of eight applications of four drops of a 0.8% solution in mineral oil produced one melanoma among 25 survivors at 33 weeks (Shubik et al., 1960).

Guinea pig: A very few experiments for skin carcinogenesis in guinea pigs have been reported. In one of them "traces" of papillomas were observed in an unspecified number of animals painted twice weekly with a 1% solution of B(a)P in benzene for over two years (Oberling et al., 1937).

Rabbit: Twice-weekly painting with a 0.3% solution of B(a)P in benzene for 400 days produced one carcinoma and 10 papillomas among 10 rabbits (Schürch & Winterstein, 1935). This result has been confirmed repeatedly (Hartwell, 1951; Thompson & Co., 1971; Tracor/Jitco, 1973a,b). Some evidence of a dose-response relationship stems from a study on small groups of rabbits painted five times weekly with concentrations of B(a)P in acetone ranging between 0.0001% and 0.5%: tumours appeared following application of concentrations of 0.005% or more (Wynder et al., 1957).

(c) <u>Inhalation and/or intratracheal administration</u>

Rat: In an inhalation study, of a group of 21 rats exposed to a mixture of 10 mg/m^3 B(a)P + 3.5 ppm SO_2 for one hour/day for more than a year, two developed squamous cell carcinomas of the lung. In another group of 21 rats which received an additional treatment with SO_2 of 10 ppm for six hours/day, squamous cell carcinomas appeared in five rats. No tumours were found among three rats receiving SO_2 only. No group was exposed to B(a)P alone (Laskin et al., 1970).

The production of lung tumours following intratracheal administration of B(a)P was first demonstrated by Ryazanov et al. (1961) in a study in which one or five intratracheal administrations of 100 mg B(a)P to eight rats produced at least three lung tumours. In a more recent dose-response study, 10 monthly intratracheal injections of either 0.0005, 0.002, 0.01, 0.05, 0.25 or 2.5 mg B(a)P mixed with a blood substitute, BK-8, and India ink were followed by an observation period of about a further two years. No lung tumours were found at the two lowest concentrations, while at higher dosages percentages of animals developing lung tumours were, respectively, 14%, 28%, 43% and 80% (Yanisheva, 1971).

Hamster: In an inhalation study, hamsters exposed to mixtures of B(a)P and SO_2, in a schedule similar to that indicated above for rats, died relatively early without neoplastic changes (Laskin et al., 1970). In another experiment, tracheal papillomas and carcinomas were observed in hamsters exposed to approximately 2.5 mg B(a)P as a spray in sesame oil thrice weekly for one year (Mohr, 1971).

The induction of bronchial tumours in hamsters following intratracheal injections of B(a)P was first demonstrated by Herrold & Dunham (1962): weekly instillations of 0.5 mg B(a)P in Tween 60 for five to six months produced a total of five tracheobronchial tumours in three animals out of five surviving for nine months. In other studies, it was observed that weekly doses of aqueous colloidal suspensions of B(a)P did not produce tumours (Laskin et al., 1970). On the contrary, a model for the induction of bronchogenic carcinomas was found to be repeated instillations of a saline suspension of a dust containing fine crystalline particles of B(a)P attached by surface adhesion to fine particles of ferric oxide (Saffiotti et al., 1968). A dose-response study with weekly intratracheal administrations of equal amounts of B(a)P and ferric oxide failed to demonstrate a no-effect level, as the lowest dose used, 0.25 mg B(a)P/week, produced one tumour of the respiratory tract in each of 10/88 hamsters. The highest dose used was 3 mg B(a)P/week, and this produced a total of 58 tumours of the respiratory tract in 34/57 hamsters (Saffiotti et al., 1972). On the other hand, in the same experimental system with 20 weekly doses of 0.5 mg/week, B(a)P was less effective than 7H-dibenzo(c,g)carbazole, since the former induced tumours of the respiratory tract in 30% of the animals and the latter did so in 89% (Sellakumar & Shubik, 1972).

Duck: Thirty-four ducks were given a single intratracheal dose of 50-200 mg B(a)P in Tween 80. Survival rate was poor. One animal developed a lung carcinoma and two had bronchial squamous metaplasia (Rigdon & Neal, 1965).

Monkey: In a study still in progress at the time of reporting, weekly intratracheal instillations of 3-15 mg B(a)P with an equivalent amount of ferric oxide induced squamous carcinomas of the lung in at least two of an original number of six subhuman primates, Galago crassicaudatus (Crocker et al., 1970).

(d) Subcutaneous and/or intramuscular administration

Mouse: Many studies on the subcutaneous carcinogenicity of B(a)P have been carried out (Hartwell, 1951; Shubik & Hartwell, 1957, 1969; Thompson & Co., 1971; Tracor/Jitco, 1973a,b). Several dose-response studies are available, some of which permit a comparison with other carcinogens tested under the same conditions in the same laboratory. In the work of Bryan & Shimkin (1943) on the induction of local sarcomas following single injections of B(a)P in tricaprylin, no tumours were found following doses of 0.031 mg or less, whereas four of 20 C3H mice developed tumours with 0.062 mg, and higher tumour incidences were obtained following greater doses. The thresholds of carcinogenicity for 3-methylcholanthrene (MC) and dibenz(a,h)anthracene (DB(a,h)A) in the same experiment were, respectively, 0.0078 and 0.0019 mg. However, the average minimal latent periods were three months for B(a)P, two-and-a-half months for MC and 3.7 months for DB(a,h)A.

In a more recent dose-response study on C57 mice in which a 1:9 cholesterol:olive oil mixture was used as the solvent, 0.00004 mg were ineffective, whereas 0.0004, 0.004 and 0.04 mg produced sarcomas in, respectively, one, five and 23 mice of groups of 50 (Hieger, 1959). In a further study on CFW Swiss mice, B(a)P in cottonseed oil produced no tumours at doses of 0.001-0.01 mg, while 0.025 mg or more were effective (Rigdon & Neal, 1971).

Newborn mouse: Induction of hepatomas and/or lung adenomas and occasional tumours at other sites in mice of different strains was recorded following administrations of B(a)P during the first days of life at doses of 20-40 µg/mouse in different solvents (Pietra et al., 1961; Roe & Waters, 1967; Tóth & Shubik, 1967; Grant et al., 1968).

Rat: Among the many positive experiments, only a study by Oberling et al. (1939) was dose-response designed. Single injections of 0.05, 0.1, 0.5 and

1 mg B(a)P in olive oil produced tumours, respectively, in 1/7, 4/31, 9/17 and 64/69 rats.

Hamster: Injections of 2.5 mg B(a)P produced sarcomas in 37 of 40 animals, with a latent period of 140-150 days (Halberstaedter, 1969). This was confirmed in subsequent studies. Only one dose-response study is available: groups of 12 hamsters were given a single subcutaneous injection of B(a)P in heated olive oil; none and one tumour were produced by 0.005 and 0.01 mg respectively. The percentage of animals bearing tumours approached 100% at 1 mg and above (Rivière et al., 1963).

Guinea pig: An injection of 5 mg B(a)P in lard to four guinea pigs induced tumours in all animals within 394 days (Haagensen & Krehbiel, 1936). This was confirmed in other studies (Shear, 1938).

Rabbit: Negative results have been obtained in a few experiments on small numbers of animals (Hartwell, 1951; Shubik & Hartwell, 1957, 1969; Thompson & Co., 1971; Tracor/Jitco, 1973a,b).

Newt: Single injections of 10-400 µg B(a)P were given to a total of 160 Triturus cristatus which were then sacrificed at intervals up to one year after treatment. Tumours were observed in animals given more than 20 µg (Seilern-Aspang & Kratochwil, 1962).

Monkey: A metastatizing and transplantable sarcoma at the site of injection appeared within six months after administration of 10 mg B(a)P in olive oil to one tree shrew, Tupaia glis (Noyes, 1968). A similar observation was made in the cottontop marmoset, Saguinus oedipus, although the latent period was longer (Noyes, 1969).

(e) Intraperitoneal administrttion

Mouse: Weekly i.p. injections of 2 mg B(a)P as a colloidal suspension in water to 80 ST/A mice induced abdominal fibrosarcomas in 81% of 40 females and 73% of 40 males with an average latent period of 33 weeks (Payne, 1958).

Rat: A single i.p. administration of 10 mg B(a)P produced two mammary and two uterine carcinomas among 10 Wistar rats within one year, whereas no mammary tumours were found in the controls (Payne, 1958).

(f) Other experimental systems:

Intravenous injection: A dose of 39 mg/kg in lipid emulsion given intravenously to 50-day-old female Sprague Dawley rats induced mammary carcinomas in nine of 30 animals within 98 days (Pataki & Huggins, 1969).

Intrabronchial implantation: Following intrabronchial implantation to rats of 3-5 mg pellets containing B(a)P in cholesterol at concentrations ranging from 0.1-100%, borderline activity was detected at concentrations of 0.1 and 1%, while sizable incidences of tumours were produced by pellets containing 10% B(a)P or more. Incidences were dose-related and reached a maximum of about 25% following implantation of pellets containing 100% B(a)P (Laskin et al., 1970).

Transplacental route: Three s.c. or i.p. injections to ICR/Ha mice of 2-4 mg B(a)P at the 11th, 13th and 15th day of pregnancy resulted in an increased incidence of lung adenomas and initiation of skin carcinogenesis in the offspring (Bulay & Wattenberg, 1970; Bulay, 1970). Foster nursing did not alter these effects (Bulay & Wattenberg, 1971).

B(a)P has proved to be carcinogenic in a variety of other experimental systems such as lung fixation, implantation in the stomach wall, renal parenchyma, brain and other organs, injection into the renal pelvis, vaginal painting etc. (Hartwell, 1951; Shubik,& Hartwell, 1957, 1969; Thompson & Co., 1971; Tracor/Jitco, 1973a,b).

3.2 Other relevant biological data

(a) Animals

The hepatobiliary system and the gastrointestinal tract are the main routes of elimination of B(a)P and its metabolites in different species, independent of the route of administration (Peacock, 1936). That the liver metabolism plays a role in local carcinogenesis has been suggested by experiments in which subcutaneous sarcomas following B(a)P injection occurred to a greater extent in mice in which liver injury was produced with carbon tetrachloride than it did in the controls (Kotin et al., 1962).

Several studies carried out in different experimental systems (including in vitro studies) have revealed the presence in the liver, in the bile and in the intestine of primary and secondary oxidation products. The main metabolites are 3- and 6-hydroxyB(a)P and some dihydro-dihydroxy derivatives (Berenblum & Schoental, 1943a;

Falk et al., 1962; Sims, 1967, 1970a,b). The absence among the latter of dihydrodiols in the K-region has been emphasized (Sims, 1970a,b).

(<u>b</u>) <u>Man</u>

No data on B(a)P metabolism in man is available. Human lung tissue and lymph nodes from the tracheobronchial region were found to contain B(a)P (Perdriau, 1963; Sula, 1963). Cultures of human epidermal cells exhibit a toxic response in the presence of B(a)P, suggesting that the cells possess a microsomal aryl hydrolase system which is capable of converting the hydrocarbon into a toxic metabolite (Dietz & Flaxman, 1971). Primary embryonic human lung cells resembled mouse embryo cells in the degree to which B(a)P was bound to cellular macromolecules following metabolism (Brookes & Duncan, 1971).

(<u>c</u>) <u>Carcinogenicity of metabolites</u>

Some of the hydroxyderivatives of B(a)P have been tested for carcinogenicity by subcutaneous injection or skin painting with negative results (Berenblum & Schoental, 1943a; Harper, 1957, 1958). However in a recent experiment on rats, B(a)P and 6-hydroxymethylB(a)P exhibited a similar ability to induce local sarcomas (Flesher & Sydnor, 1973).

3.3 <u>Observations in man</u>

Only a few reports on the effects on man of B(a)P are available. Regressing verrucae developed in all 26 patients who were given up to 120 skin applications of a 1% solution of B(a)P in benzene over a period of four months in apparently healthy areas of the body (Cottini & Mazzone, 1939). Similar changes were mentioned in another report concerning accidental exposure to B(a)P (Rhoads et al., 1954). A persistent nodule which was histologically diagnosed as squamous epithelioma developed in a man who had been exposed to B(a)P for three weeks while he was carrying out an experiment in mice (Klar, 1938).

4. Comments on Data Reported and Evaluation

4.1 Animal data

B(a)P has produced tumours in all of the nine species for which data are reported following different administrations including oral, skin and intratracheal routes. It has both a local and a systemic carcinogenic effect. In sub-human primates, there is convincing evidence of the ability of B(a)P to produce local sarcomas following repeated subcutaneous injections and lung carcinomas following intratracheal instillation. It is also an initiator of skin carcinogenesis in mice, and it is carcinogenic in single-dose experiments and following prenatal exposure.

In skin carcinogenesis studies in mice B(a)P was consistently found to produce more tumours in a shorter period of time than did other polycyclic aromatic hydrocarbons, with the possible exception of DB(a,h)A (see other monographs published in this volume). In a dose-response study involving subcutaneous injection in mice, the minimal dose at which carcinogenicity was detected was higher for B(a)P than for DB(a,h)A and for MC. However, the latent periods were shorter for B(a)P than for DB(a,h)A. In studies using intratracheal administration, B(a)P appeared to be less effective than 7H-dibenzo(c,g)carbazole in the hamster.

4.2 Human data

No epidemiological studies on the significance of B(a)P exposure to man are available, and the studies reported in section 3.3 are insufficient to prove that B(a)P is carcinogenic for man. However, coal-tar and other materials which are known to be carcinogenic to man may contain B(a)P. The substance has also been detected in other environmental situations. The possible contribution of polycyclic aromatic hydrocarbons from some environmental sources to the overall carcinogenic risk to man is discussed in the preamble.

Similarities of metabolism of B(a)P in human and mouse cells cultured *in vitro* have been reported. The relevance of this finding for evaluating the risk for man cannot yet be assessed.

5. References

Allsopp, C.B. (1940) Photo-oxides of carcinogenic hydrocarbons. Nature (Lond.), 145, 303

Andelman, J.B. & Suess, N.J. (1970) Polynuclear aromatic hydrocarbons in the water environment. Bull. Wld Hlth Org., 43, 479

Badger, G.M., Donnelly, J.K. & Spotswood, T.M. (1964) The formation of aromatic hydrocarbons at high temperatures. XIII. The pyrolysis of anthracene. Aust. J. Chem., 17, 1147

Badger, G.M., Donnelly, J.K. & Spotswood, T.M. (1965) The formation of aromatic hydrocarbons at high temperatures. XXIV. The pyrolysis of some tobacco constituents. Aust. J. Chem., 18, 1249

Bailey, E.J. & Dungal, N. (1958) Polycyclic hydrocarbons in Icelandic smoked food. Brit. J. Cancer, 12, 348

Bartle, K.D., Jones, D.W. & Matthews, R.S. (1969) High-field nuclear magnetic resonance spectra of some carcinogenic polynuclear hydrocarbons. Spectrochim. Acta, 25A, 1603

Beilsteins Handbuch der Organischen Chemie, 5, III, 2517

Berenblum, I. & Schoental, R. (1943a) The metabolism of 3,4-benzpyrene in mice and rats. I. The isolation of a hydroxy and a quinone derivative, and a consideration of their biological significance. Cancer Res., 3, 145

Berenblum, I. & Schoental, R. (1943b) Carcinogenic constituents of shale oil. Brit. J. exp. Path., 24, 232

Berner, G. & Biernoth, G. (1969) Über den Gehalt erhitzter Öle und Fette an polycyclischen aromatischen Kohlenwasserstoffen. Z. Lebensmitt.-Untersuch., 140, 330

Bhatia, K. (1971) Gas chromatographic determination of polycyclic aromatic hydrocarbons. Analyt. Chem., 43, 609

Biernoth, G. & Rost, H.E. (1967) The occurrence of polycyclic aromatic hydrocarbons in coconut oil and their removal. Chem. and Ind., 2002

Biernoth, G. & Rost, H.E. (1968) Vorkommen polycyclischer aromatischer Kohlenwasserstoffe in Speiseölen und deren Entfernung. Arch. Hyg. (Muenchen), 152, 238

Bingham, E. & Falk, H.L. (1969) Environmental carcinogens. The modifying effect of cocarcinogens on the threshold response. Arch. environ. Hlth, 19, 779

Blumer, M. (1961) Benzpyrenes in soil. Science, 134, 474

Bonnet, J. (1962) Quantitative analysis of benzo(a)pyrene in vapors coming from melted tar. Nat. Cancer Inst. Monogr., 9, 221

Borneff, J. & Fábián, B. (1966) Kanzerogene Substanzen in Speisefett und -öl. Arch. Hyg. (Muenchen), 150, 485

Borneff, J. & Fischer, R. (1962) Kanzerogene Substanzen in Wasser und Boden. IX. Polyzyclische, aromatische Kohlenwasserstoffe in Walderde. Arch. Hyg. (Muenchen), 146, 430

Borneff, J. & Kunte, H. (1963) Kanzerogene Substanzen in Wasser und Boden. XIV. Weitere Untersuchungen über polyzyclische aromatische Kohlenwasserstoffe in Erdproben. Arch. Hyg. (Muenchen), 147, 401

Borneff, J. & Kunte, H. (1964) Kanzerogene Substanzen in Wasser und Boden. XVI. Nachweis von polyzyklischen Aromaten in Wasserproben durch direkte Extraktion. Arch. Hyg. (Muenchen), 148, 585

Borneff, J. & Kunte, H. (1965) Kanzerogene Substanzen in Wasser und Boden. XVII. Über die Herkunft und Bewertung der polyzyklischen, aromatischen Kohlenwasserstoffe im Wasser. Arch. Hyg. (Muenchen), 149, 226

Borneff, J. & Kunte, H. (1967) Kanzerogene Substanzen in Wasser und Boden. XIX. Wirkung der Abwasserreinigung auf polyzyklische Aromaten. Arch. Hyg. (Muenchen), 151, 202

Borneff, J. & Kunte, H. (1969) Kanzerogene Substanzen in Wasser und Boden. XXVI. Routine methode zur Bestimmung von polyzyklischen Aromaten im Wasser. Arch. Hyg. (Muenchen), 153, 220

Borneff, J., Selenka, F., Kunte, H. & Maximos, A. (1968) Experimental studies on the formation of polycyclic aromatic hydrocarbons in plants. Environ. Res., 2, 22

Bosco, G., Barsini, G. & Grella, A. (1967) Nuove indagini sulla presenza di idrocarburi policiclici aromatici nel pulviscolo atmosferico del centro storico della citta di Siena. Arch. environ. Hlth, 14, 285

Boyland, E. (1933) Inhibition of lactic dehydrogenase by derivatives of carcinogenic compounds. Biochem. J., 27, 971

Boyland, E. & Green, B. (1962a) The interaction of polycyclic hydrocarbons and nucleic acids. Brit. J. Cancer, 16, 507

Boyland, E. & Green, B. (1962b) The interaction of polycyclic hydrocarbons and purines. Brit. J. Cancer, 16, 347

Brookes, P. & Duncan, M.E. (1971) Carcinogenic hydrocarbons and human cells in culture. Nature (Lond.), 234, 40

Bryan, W.R. & Shimkin, M.B. (1943) Quantitative analysis of dose-response data obtained with three carcinogenic hydrocarbons in strain C3H male mice. J. nat Cancer Inst., 3, 503

Bulay, O.M. (1970) The study of development of lung and skin tumours in mice exposed in vitro to polycyclic hydrocarbons. Acta med. Turc., 7, 3

Bulay, O.M. & Wattenberg, L.W. (1970) Carcinogenic effect of subcutaneous administration of benzo(a)pyrene during pregnancy on the progeny. Proc. Soc. exp. Biol. (N.Y.), 135, 84

Bulay, O.M. & Wattenberg, L.W. (1971) Carcinogenic effects of polycyclic hydrocarbon carcinogen administration to mice during pregnancy on the progeny. J. nat. Cancer Inst., 46, 397

Chu, E.W. & Malmgren, R.A. (1965) An inhibitory effect of vitamin A on the induction of tumors of forestomach and cervix in the Syrian hamster by carcinogenic polycyclic hydrocarbons. Cancer Res., 25, 884

Clar, E. (1964) Polycyclic Hydrocarbons, Vol. 2, London, New York, Academic Press; Berlin, Göttingen, Heidelberg, Springer-Verlag, p. 130

Cleary, G.J. (1963) Measurement of polycyclic aromatic hydrocarbons in the air of Sydney using very long alumina columns for separation. Int. J. air wat. Pollut., 7, 753

Cleary, G.J. & Sullivan, J.L. (1965) Pollution by polycyclic aromatic hydrocarbons in the city of Sydney. Med. J. Aust., 1, 758

Colucci, J.M. & Begeman, C.R. (1965) The automotive contribution to air-borne polynuclear aromatic hydrocarbons in Detroit. J. air Pollut. Control Ass., 15, 113

Commins, B.T. & Waller, R.E. (1967) Observations from a ten-year study of pollution at a site in the city of London. Atmosph. Environ., 1, 49

Conlee, C.J., Kenline, P.A., Cummins, R.L. & Konopinski, V.J. (1967) Motor vehicle exhaust at three selected sites. Arch. environ. Hlth, 14, 429

Cook, J.W. (1933) The production of cancer by pure chemical compounds. In: Torre Blanco, J. & Wissmann, S.C., eds., Congreso Internacional de Lucha Cientifica y Social contra el Cancer, Madrid, Vol. 2, Madrid, Blass, p. 373

Cook, J.W., Hewett, C.L. & Hieger, I. (1933) The isolation of a cancer-producing hydrocarbon from coal-tar. J. chem. Soc., 395

Cottini, G.B. & Mazzone, G.B. (1939) The effects of 3,4-benzpyrene on human skin. Amer. J. Cancer, 37, 186

Crocker, T.T., Chase, J.E., Wells, S.A. & Nunes, L.L. (1970) Preliminary report on experimental squamous carcinoma of the lung in hamsters and in a primate (Galago Crassicaudatus). In: Nettesheim, P., Hanna, M.G. & Deatherage, J.W., eds., Morphology of Experimental Respiratory Carcinogenesis (US Atomic Energy Commission Symposium Series No. 21), p. 317

Davis, W.W., Krahl, M.E. & Clowes, G.H.A. (1942) Solubility of carcinogenic and related hydrocarbons in water. J. amer. chem. Soc., 64, 108

Del Vecchio, V., Valori, P., Melchiorri, C. & Grella, A. (1970) Aromatic hydrocarbons from gasoline-engine and liquefied petroleum gas engine exhausts. Pure appl. Chem., 24, 739

DeMaio, L. & Corn, M. (1966) Polynuclear aromatic hydrocarbons associated with particulates in Pittsburgh air. J. air Pollut. Control Ass., 16, 67

Dietz, M.H. & Flaxman, B.A. (1971) Toxicity of aromatic hydrocarbons on normal human epidermal cells in vitro. Cancer Res., 31, 1206

Dikun, P.P. & Nikberg, J.J. (1958) Study of air pollution with 3,4-benzopyrene in the area of an old type coal-processing plant. Vop. Onkol., 4, 669

Dontenwill, W. & Mohr, U. (1962) Experimentelle Untersuchungen zum Problem der carcinomentstehung im Respirationstrakt. I. Die unterschiedlicke Wirkung des Benzpyrens auf die Epithelien der Haut, der Mundhöhle und der Trachea des Goldhamsters. Z. Krebsforsch., 65, 56

Dungal, N. (1959) Können geräuchte Speisen krebserzeugend sein. Krebsarzt, 14, 22

Edstrom, T. & Petro, B.A. (1968) Gel permeation chromatographic studies of polynuclear aromatic hydrocarbon materials. J. polymer Sci. C, 21, 171

Eisenbrand, J. & Baumann, K. (1970) Über die Erhöhung der Wasserlöslichkeit von 3,4-Benzpyren durch Zusatz von 1,3,7-Trimethylxanthin (Coffein). IV, V. Dtsch. Lebensmitt.-Rdsch., 66, 297, 430

Elmenhorst, H. & Grimmer, G. (1968) Polycyclische Kohlenwasserstoffe aus Zigarettenrauchkondensat. Eine Methode zur Fraktionierung grosser Mengen für Tierversuche. Z. Krebsforsch., 71, 66

Epstein, S.S., Joshi, S., Andrea, J., Mantel, N., Sawicki, E., Stanley, T. & Tabor, E.C. (1966) Carcinogenicity of organic particulate pollutants in urban air after administration of trace quantities to neonatal mice. Nature(Lond.), 212, 1305

Fábián, B. (1968) Kanzerogene Substanzen in Speisefett und -öl. IV. Untersuchungen an Margarine, Pflanzenfett und Butter. Arch. Hyg. (Muenchen), 152, 231

Fábián, B. (1969) Kanzerogene Substanzen in Speisefett und -öl. VI. Weitere Untersuchungen an Margarine und Schokolade. Arch. Hyg. (Muenchen), 153, 21

Falk, H.L., Steiner, P., Goldfein, S., Breslow, A. & Hykes, R. (1951) Carcinogenic hydrocarbons and related compounds in processed rubber. Cancer Res., 11, 318

Falk, H.L., Kotin, P. & Markul, I. (1958) The disappearance of carcinogens from soot in human lungs. Cancer, 11, 482

Falk, H.L., Kotin, P., Lee, S.S. & Nathan, A. (1962) Intermediary metabolism of benzo(a)pyrene in the rat. J. nat. Cancer Inst., 28, 699

Fischer, R. (1970) Spektrophotometrisches Verfahren zur raschen Beurteilung von Russen auf ihren Gehalt an polycyclischen, aromatischen Kohlenwasserstoffen. Z. analyt. Chem., 249, 110

Flesher, J.W. & Sydnor, K.L. (1973) Possible role of 6-hydroxymethylbenzo(a)pyrene as a proximate carcinogen of benzo(a)pyrene and 6-methylbenzo(a)pyrene. Int. J. Cancer, 11, 433

Fritz, W. (1966) Polycyclische aromatische Kohlenwasser in Malzkaffee, Gerste und Malz. Naturwissenschaften, 53, 132

Fritz, W. (1968a) 3,4-Benzpyren und andere Polyaromaten in Margarine und Mayonaise. Nahrung, 12, 495

Fritz, W. (1968b) Zur Bildung cancerogener Kohlenwasserstoffe bei der thermischen Behandlung von Lebensmitteln. II. Das Rösten von Bohnenkaffee und Kaffee-Ersatzstoffen. Nahrung, 12, 799

Fritz, W. (1968c) Zur Bildung cancerogener Kohlenwasserstoffe bei der thermischen Behandlung von Lebensmitteln. III. Das Backen von Brot und Biskuits. Nahrung, 12, 805

Fritz, W. (1968d) Zur Bildung cancerogener Kohlenwasserstoffe bei der thermischen Behandlung von Lebensmitteln. IV. Der Einfluss des Frittierens. Nahrung, 12, 809

Fritz, W. (1969) Zur Lösungsverhalten der Polyaromaten beim Kochen von Kaffee-Ersatzstoffen und Bohnenkaffee. Dtsch. Lebensmitt.-Rdsch., 65, 83

Fritz, W. & Engst, R. (1971) Zur umweltbedingten Kontamination von Lebensmitteln mit krebserzeugenden Kohlenwasserstoffen. Z. ges. Hyg., 17, 271

Fryčka, J. (1972) Separation of polynuclear aromatic hydrocarbons by gas-solid chromatography on graphitized carbon black deposited on chromosorb W. J. Chromat., 65, 432

Gibel, W. (1964) Experimenteller Beitrag zur Synkarzinogenese beim Speiseröhrenkarzinom. Krebsarzt, 19, 268

Gilbert, J.A.S. & Lindsey, A.J. (1957) The thermal decomposition of some tobacco constituents. Brit. J. Cancer, 11, 398

Gladen, R. (1972) The determination of carcinogenic polycyclic aromatic hydrocarbons in automobile exhaust gases by column chromatography. Chromatographia, 5, 236

Gorelova, N.D., Dikun, P.P., Solinek, V.A. & Emshanova, A.V. (1960) The content of 3,4-benzpyrene in fish smoked by different methods. Vop. Onkol., 6, 39

Gouw, T.H., Whittemore, I.M. & Jentoft, R.E. (1970) Versatile short capillary column in gas chromatography. Analyt. Chem., 42, 1394

Gräf, W. & Diehl, H. (1966) Über den naturbedingten Normalpegel kanzerogener polycyclischer Aromate und seine Ursache. Arch. Hyg. (Muenchen), 150, 49

Grant, G.A., Carter, R.L., Roe, F.J.C. & Pike, M.C. (1968) Effects of the neonatal injection of a carcinogen on the induction of tumours by the subsequent application to the skin of the same carcinogen. Brit. J. Cancer, 22, 346

Grimmer, G. (1961) Eine Methode zur Bestimmung von 3,4-Benzpyren in Tabakrauchkondensaten. Beitr. Tabakforsch., 1, 107

Grimmer, G. (1966) Cancerogene Kohlenwasserstoffe in der Umgebung des Menschen. Erdöl Kohle-Erdgas-Petrochem., 19, 578

Grimmer, G. & Düvel, D. (1970) Untersuchungen zur endogenen Bildung von polycyclischen Kohlenwasserstoffen in höheren Pflanzen. 8. Cancerogene Kohlenwasserstoffe in der Umgebung des Menschen. Z. Naturforsch., 25B, 1171

Grimmer, G. & Hildebrandt, A. (1965a) Kohlenwasserstoffe in der Umgebung des Menschen. II. Der Gehalt polycyclishcer Kohlenwasserstoffe in Brotgetreide verschiedener Standorte. Z. Krebsforsch., 67, 272

Grimmer, G. & Hildebrandt, A. (1965b) Kohlenwasserstoffe in der Umgebung des Menschen. III. Der Gehalt polycyclischer Kohlenwasserstoffe in verschiedenen Gemüsesorten und Salaten. Dtsch. Lebensmitt.-Rdsch., 61, 272

Grimmer, G. & Hildebrandt, A. (1966) Der Gehalt polycyclischer Kohlenwasserstoffe in Kaffee und Tee. Dtsch. Lebensmitt.-Rdsch., 62, 19

Grimmer, G. & Hildebrandt, A. (1967a) Kohlenwasserstoffe in der Umgebung des Menschen. V. Der Gehalt polycyclischer Kohlenwasserstoffe in Fleisch und Räucherwaren. Z. Krebsforsch., 69, 223

Grimmer, G. & Hildebrandt, A. (1967b) Content of polycyclic hydrocarbons in crude vegetable oils. Chem. and Ind., 2000

Grimmer, G. & Wilhelm, G. (1969) Der Gehalt von polycyclischen Kohlenwasserstoffen in europäischen Hefen. Dtsch. Lebensmitt.-Rdsch., 65, 229

Grimmer, G., Jacob, J. & Hildebrandt, A. (1972) Kohlenwasserstoffe in der Umgebung des Menschen. IX. Der Gehalt polycyclischer Kohlenwasserstoffe in isländischen Bodenproben. Z. Krebsforsch., 78, 65

Grushko, I.M., Dikun, P.P., Shabad, Y.M., Sukavishnikova, T.J., Zak, L.M. & Vlassenko, O.M. (1958) Study of air pollution with 3,4-benzopyrene in Angarsk and Irkutsk. Gig. i Sanit., 4, 7

Haagensen, C.D. & Krehbiel, O.F. (1936) Liposarcoma produced by 1,2-benzpyrene. Amer. J. Cancer, 27, 474

Haigh, C.W., Mallion, R.B. & Armour, E.A.G. (1970) Proton magnetic resonance of planar condensed benzenoid hydrocarbons. II. A critical evaluation of the McWeeny 'ring current' theory. Molec. Phys., 18, 751

Halberstaedter, L. (1939) A benzpyrene tumour strain in hamsters with tendency to metastasis formation. Nature (Lond.), 144, 377

Hamm, R. & Tóth, L. (1970) Cancerogene Kohlenwasserstoffe in geräucherten Fleischerzeugnissen. Med. u. Ernähr, 11, 25

Hangebrauck, R.P., von Lehmden, D.J. & Meeker, J.E. (1964) Emissions of polynuclear hydrocarbons and other pollutants from heat-generation and incineration processes. J. air Pollut. Control Ass., 14, 267

Hangebrauck, R.P., Lauch, R.P. & Meeker, J.E. (1966) Emissions of polynuclear hydrocarbons from automobiles and trucks. Am. industr. Hyg. Ass. J., 27, 47

Harington, J.S. (1962) Occurrence of oils containing 3,4-benzopyrene and related substances in asbestos. Nature (Lond.), 193, 43

Harper, K.H. (1957) The carcinogenicity of benzpyrene metabolites. A. R. Brit. Emp. Cancer Campgn, 35, 151

Harper, K.H. (1958) The carcinogenicity of benzopyrene metabolites. A. R. Brit. Emp. Cancer Campgn, 36, 180

Hartwell, J.L. (1951) Survey of compounds which have been tested for carcinogenic activity, Washington, D.C., Government Printing Office (Public Health Service Publication No. 149)

Herrold, K.M. & Dunham, L.J. (1962) Induction of carcinoma and papilloma of the tracheobronchial mucosa of the Syrian hamster by intratracheal instillation of benzo(a)pyrene. J. nat. Cancer Inst., 28, 467

Hettche, H.O. (1971) Plant waxes as collectors of polycyclic aromatics in the air of residential areas. Staub (Engl. Transl.), 31, 34

Hieger, I. (1959) Carcinogenesis by cholesterol. Brit. J. Cancer, 13, 439

Hoffmann, D. & Wynder, E.L. (1962a) A study of air pollution carcinogenesis. II. The isolation and identification of polynuclear aromatic hydrocarbons from gasoline engine exhaust condensate. Cancer, 15, 93

Hoffmann, D. & Wynder, E.L. (1962b) Analytical and biological studies on gasoline engine exhaust. Nat. Cancer Inst. Monogr., 9, 91

Hoffmann, D. & Wynder, E.L. (1963) Studies on gasoline engine exhaust. J. air Pollut. Control Ass., 13, 322

Hoffmann, D. & Wynder, E.L. (1966) Beitrag zur carcinogenen Wirkung von Dibenzopyrenen. Z. Krebsforsch., 68, 137

Hood, L.V. & Winefordner, J.D. (1968) Thin-layer separation and low-temperature luminescence measurement of mixtures of carcinogens. Analyt. Chim. Acta, 42, 199

Howard, J.W., Teague, R.T., White, R.H. & Fry, B.E. (1966a) Extraction and estimation of polycyclic aromatic hydrocarbons in smoked foods. I. General method. J. Ass. off. analyt. Chem., 49, 595

Howard, J.W., Turicchi, E.W., White, R.H. & Fazio, T. (1966b) Extraction and estimation of polycyclic aromatic hydrocarbons in vegetable oils. J. Ass. off. analyt. Chem., 49, 1236

Huggins, C. & Yang, N.C. (1962) Induction and extinction of mammary cancer. Science, 137, 257

Jung, L. & Morand, P. (1963) Présence de pyrène, de benzo-1,2-pyrène et de benzo-3,4-pyrène dans différentes huiles végetales. C.R. Acad. Sci. (Paris), 257, 1638

Klar, E. (1938) Über die Entstehung eines Epithelioms beim Menschen nach experimentellen Arbeiten mit Benzpyren. Klin. Wschr., 17, 1279

Klimisch, H.J. & Reese, D. (1972) Das gelchromatographische Trennverhalten von Polystyrolgel für Kohlenwasserstoffe, Amine und Phenole. Präparative Fraktionierung von Cigarettenrauchkondensat für biologische Versuche. J. Chromat., 67, 299

Kotin, P. & Falk, H.L. (1963) Atmospheric factors in pathogenesis of lung cancer. Advanc. Cancer Res., 7, 475

Kotin, P., Falk, H.L. & Miller, A. (1962) Effect of carbon tetrachloride intoxication on metabolism of benzo(a)-pyrene in rats and mice. J. nat. Cancer Inst., 28, 725

Kreyberg, L. (1959) 3,4-Benzpyrene in industrial air pollution: some reflexions. Brit. J. Cancer, 13, 618

Kroeller, E. (1965a) Ergebnisse von Schwelversuchen an Zusatzstoffen zu Tabakwaren. 3. Pflanzliche Schleim-und Gummiarten. Dtsch. Lebensmitt.-Rdsch., 65, 150

Kroeller, E. (1965b) Ergebnisse von Schwelversuchen an Zusatzstoffen zu Tabakwaren. 2. Polyglykole, glycerin. Dtsch. Lebensmitt.-Rdsch., 61, 16

Kronberger, H. & Weiss, J. (1944) Formation and structure of some organic molecular compounds. III. The dielectric polarisation of some solid crystalline molecular compounds. J. chem. Soc., 146, 464

Kuratsune, M. & Hueper, W.C. (1960) Polycyclic aromatic hydrocarbons in roasted coffee. J. nat. Cancer Inst., 24, 463

Lam, J. (1956a) Isolation and identification of 3,4-benzpyrene, chrysene, and a number of other aromatic hydrocarbons in the pyrolysis products from dicetyl. Acta path. microbiol. scand., 39, 198

Lam, J. (1956b) Determination of 3,4-benzpyrene and other aromatic compounds formed by pyrolysis of aliphatic tobacco hydrocarbons. Acta path. microbiol. scand., 39, 207

Laskin, S., Kuschner, M. & Drew, R.T. (1970) Studies in pulmonary carcinogenesis. In: Hanna, M.G., Nettesheim, P. & Gilbert, J.R., eds., Inhalation Carcinogenesis (US Atomic Energy Commission Symposium Series No. 18), p. 321

Lawther, P.J., Commins, B.T. & Waller, R.E. (1965) A study of the concentrations of polycyclic aromatic hydrocarbons in gas works retort houses. Brit. J. industr. Med., 22, 13.

Lijinsky, W. & Raha, C.R. (1961) Polycyclic aromatic hydrocarbons in commercial solvents. Toxicol. appl. Pharmacol., 3, 469

Lijinsky, W. & Ross, A.E. (1967) Production of carcinogenic polynuclear hydrocarbons in the cooking of food. Food cosmet. Toxicol., 5, 343

Lijinsky, W. & Shubik, P. (1964) Benzo(a)pyrene and other polynuclear hydrocarbons in charcoal-broiled meat. Science, 145, 53

Lijinsky, W. & Shubik, P. (1965) Polynuclear hydrocarbon carcinogens in cooked meat and smoked food. Industr. Med. Surg., 34, 152

Lijinsky, W. & Zeckmeister, L. (1953) On the catalytic hydrogenation of 3,4-benzpyrene. J. amer. chem. Soc., 75, 5495

Lijinsky, W., Domsky, I., Mason, G., Ramahi, H.Y. & Safavi, T. (1963) The chromatographic determination of trace amounts of polynuclear hydrocarbons in petrolatum, mineral oil, and coal-tar. Analyt. Chem., 35, 952

Louw, C.W. (1965) The quantitative determination of benzo(a)pyrene in the air of South African cities. Amer. industr. Hyg. Ass. J., 26, 520

Maier, von H.G. & Stender, W. (1969) Cancerogene Kohlenwasserstoffe in Kaffee-Ersatz-Produkten. Dtsch. Lebensmitt.-Rdsch., 65, 341

Malanoski, A.J., Greenfield, E.L., Barnes, C.J., Worthington, J.M. & Joe, F.L. (1968) Survey of polycyclic hydrocarbons in smoked foods. J. Ass. off. analyt. Chem., 51, 114

Mallet, L. & Héros, M. (1962) Pollution des terres végétales par les hydrocarbures polybenzéniques du type 3,4-pyrène, C.R. Acad. Sci. (Paris), 254, 958

Masek, V. (1971) Benzo(a)pyrene in the workplace atmosphere of coal and pitch coking plants. J. occup. Med., 13, 193

Masuda, Y. & Kuratsune, M. (1971) Polycyclic aromatic hydrocarbons in smoked fish, "katsuobushi". Gann, 62, 27

Masuda, Y., Mori, K., Hirohata, T. & Kuratsune, M. (1966a) Carcinogenesis in the esophagus. III. Polycyclic aromatic hydrocarbons and phenols in whisky. Gann, 57, 549

Masuda, Y., Mori, K. & Kuratsune, M. (1966b) Polycyclic aromatic hydrocarbons in common Japanese foods. I. Broiled fish, roasted barley, shoyu, and caramel. Gann, 57, 133

Masuda, Y., Mori, K. & Kuratsune, M. (1967) Polycyclic aromatic hydrocarbons formed by pyrolysis of carbohydrates, amino acids and fatty acids. Gann, 58, 69

Mecke, R. & Langenbucher, F. (1965) Infrared spectra of selected chemical compounds. London, Heiden & Son

Mohr, U. (1971) Kanzerogenese durch Diäthylnitrosamine. Untersuchungen zur diaplazentaren Wirkung. Fortschr. Med., 89, 251

Monkman, J.L., Dubois, L. & Baker, J.C. (1970) The rapid measurement of polycyclic hydrocarbons in air by microsublimation. Pure appl. Chem., 24, 731

Moriconi, E.J., Rakoczy, B. & O'Connor, W.F. (1961) Ozonolysis of polycyclic aromatics. VIII. Benzo(a)pyrene. J. amer. chem. Soc., 83, 4618

Müller, R., Moldenhauer, W. & Schlemmer, P. (1967) Erfahrungen bei der quantitativen Bestimmung von polycyclischen Kohlenwasserstoffen im Tabakrauch. Ber. Inst. Tabakforsch. (Dresden), 14, 159

Nakano, K. (1937) Experimental production of malignant tumours by 3,4-benzpyrene and 1,2,5,6-dibenzanthracene. Osaka Daig. Igaku Zassi, 36, 483

Neal, J. & Rigdon, R.H. (1967) Gastric tumors in mice fed benzo(a)pyrene: a quantitative study. Tex. Rep. Biol. Med., 25, 553

Noyes, W.F. (1968) Carcinogen-induced sarcoma in the primitive primate, Tupaia glis. Proc. Soc. exp. Biol. (N.Y.), 127, 594

Noyes, W.F. (1969) Carcinogen-induced neoplasia with metastasis in a South American primate, Saguinus oedipus. Proc. Soc. exp. Biol. (N.Y.), 131, 223

Oberling, C., Sannié, C., Guérin, M. & Guérin, P. (1937) A propos de l'action cancérigène du benzopyrène. In: Leeuwenhoek-Vereen., 5ème conference. Rapports des travaux. Amsterdam, de Bussy, p. 57

Oberling, C., Guérin, M. & Guérin, P. (1939) Particularités évolutives des tumeurs produites avec de fortes doses de benzopyrène. Bull. Ass. franç. Cancer, 28, 198

Oelert, H.H. (1969) Atypische Gelchromatographie im System Sephadex-Isopropanol. Z. analyt. Chem., 244, 91

Pataki, J. & Huggins, C. (1969) Molecular site of substituents of benz(a)anthracene related to carcinogenicity. Cancer Res., 29, 506

Payne, S. (1958) The pathological effects of the intraperitoneal injection of 3,4-benzpyrene into rats and mice. Brit. J. Cancer, 12, 65

Peacock, P.R. (1936) Evidence regarding the mechanism of elimination of 1,2-benzpyrene, 1,2,5,6-dibenzanthracene, and anthracene from the blood-stream of injected animals. Brit. J. exp. Path., 17, 164

Peirce, W.E.H. (1961) Tumour-promotion by lime oil in the mouse forestomach. Nature (Lond.), 189, 164

Perdriau, J. (1963) Pollution marine par les hydrocarbures cancérigènes type benzo-3,4 pyrène - Incidences biologiques (MD Thesis, Rouen)

Perkampus, H.H., Sandeman, I. & Timmons, C.J., eds. (1967) DMS UV Atlas of Organic Compounds, Vol. III, Weinheim, Verlag Chemie; London, Butterworths, E6/20

Pietra, G., Rappaport, H. & Shubik, P. (1961) The effects of carcinogenic chemicals in newborn mice. Cancer, 14, 308

Poel, W.E. (1959) Effect of carcinogenic dosage and duration of exposure on skin-tumour induction in mice. J. nat. Cancer Inst., 22, 19

Poel, W.E. (1963) Skin as a test site for the bioassay of carcinogens and carcinogen precursors. Nat. Cancer Inst. Monogr., 10, 611

Pouchert, C.J., ed. (1970) Aldrich Library of Infrared Spectra, Milwaukee, Wisc., Aldrich Chemical Co. Inc.

Reckner, L.R., Scott, W.E. & Biller, W.F. (1965) The composition and odor of diesel exhaust. Proc. amer. Petrol. Inst., 45, 133

Reske, G. & Stauff, J. (1963) Fluoreszenzspektren von 3,4-Benzpyren in wässrigen Medien. Z. Naturforsch., 18B, 773

Rhee, K.S. & Bratzler, L.J. (1968) Polycyclic hydrocarbon composition of wood smoke. J. food Sci., 33, 626

Rhoads, C.P., Smith, W.E., Cooper, N.S. & Sullivan, R.D. (1954) Early changes in the skins of several species, including man, after painting with carcinogenic materials. Proc. amer. Ass. Cancer Res., 1, 40

Rigdon, R.H. & Neal, J. (1965) Effect of intratracheal injection of benzo(a)pyrene on ducks. Tex. Rep. Biol. Med., 23, 494

Rigdon, R.H. & Neal, J. (1966) Gastric carcinomas and pulmonary adenomas in mice fed benzo(a)pyrene. Tex. Rep. Biol. Med., 24, 195

Rigdon, R.H. & Neal, J. (1969) Relationship of leukemia to lung and stomach tumors in mice fed benzo(a)pyrene. Proc. Soc. exp. Biol. (N.Y.), 130, 146

Rigdon, R.H. & Neal, J. (1971) Tumors in mice induced by air particulate matter from a petrochemical industrial area. Tex. Rep. Biol. Med., 29, 109

Rivière, M.R., Chouroulinkov, I. & Guérin, M. (1963) Production de tumeurs au moyen de substances chimiques cancérigènes chez le hamster. Bull. Ass. franç. Cancer, 50, 275

Roe, F.J.C. & Waters, M.A. (1967) Induction of hepatoma in mice by carcinogens of the polycyclic hydrocarbon type. Nature (Lond.), 214, 299

Roe, F.J.C., Peto, R., Kearns, F. & Bishop, D. (1970) The mechanism of carcinogenesis by the neutral fraction of cigarette smoke condensate. Brit. J. Cancer, 24, 788

Ruchkovskii, B.S., Borisyuk, Y.P., Tiktin, L.A., Popovskii, V.G., Mordkovich, M.S. & Silich, A.A. (1969) 3,4-Benzopyrene content of prunes fried by different methods. Gig. i Sanit., 34, 134

Ryazanov, V.A., Bushtueva, K.A. & Dvizhkov, P.P. (1961) Development of pulmonary cancer after intratracheal introduction of 3,4-benzpyrene. Gig. i Sanit., 26, 3

Saffiotti, U., Cefis, F. & Kolb, L.H. (1968) A method for the experimental induction of bronchogenic carcinoma. Cancer Res., 28, 104

Saffiotti, U., Montesano, R., Sellakumar, A.R. & Kaufman, D.G. (1972) Respiratory tract carcinogenesis induced in hamsters by different dose levels of benzo(a)pyrene and ferric oxide. J. nat. Cancer Inst., 49, 1199

Salaman, M.H. & Gwynn, R.H. (1951) The histology of co-carcinogenesis in mouse skin. Brit. J. Cancer, 5, 252

Sawicki, E. (1964) The separation and analysis of polynuclear aromatic hydrocarbons present in the human environment. I-III. Chemist-Analyst, 53, 24, 56, 88

Sawicki, E. (1967) Airborne carcinogens and allied compounds. Arch. environ. Hlth, 14, 46

Sawicki, E., Elbert, W., Stanley, T.W., Hauser, T.R. & Fox, F.T. (1960a) The detection and determination of polynuclear hydrocarbons in urban airborne particulates. I. The benzopyrene fraction. Int. J. air Pollut., 2, 273

Sawicki, E., Hauser, T.R. & Stanley, T.W. (1960b) Ultraviolet, visible and fluorescence spectral analysis of polynuclear hydrocarbons. Int. J. air Pollut., 2, 253

Sawicki, E., Fox, F.T., Elbert, W., Hauser, T.R. & Meeker, J. (1962a) Polynuclear aromatic hydrocarbon composition of air polluted by coal-tar pitch fumes. Amer. industr. Hyg. Ass. J., 23, 482

Sawicki, E., Hauser, T.R., Elbert, W.C., Fox, F.T. & Meeker, J.E. (1962b) Polynuclear aromatic hydrocarbon composition of the atmosphere in some large American cities. Amer. industr. Hyg. Ass. J., 23, 137

Sawicki, E., McPherson, S.P., Stanley, T.W., Meeker, J.E. & Elbert, W.C. (1965a) Quantitative composition of the urban atmosphere in terms of polynuclear aza heterocyclic compounds and aliphatic and polynuclear aromatic hydrocarbons. Int. J. air wat. Pollut., 9, 515

Sawicki, E., Meeker, J.E. & Morgan, M.J. (1965b) The quantitative composition of air pollution source effluents in terms of aza heterocyclic compounds and polynuclear aromatic hydrocarbons. Int. J. air wat. Pollut., 9, 291

Sawicki, E., Corey, R.C., Dooley, A.E., Gisclard, J.B., Monkman, J.L., Neligan, R.E. & Ripperton, L.A. (1970a) Tentative method of microanalysis for benzo(a)pyrene in airborne particulates and source effluents. Hlth lab. Sci., 7, 56

Sawicki, E., Corey, R.C., Dooley, A.E., Gisclard, J.B., Monkman, J.L., Neligan, R.E. & Ripperton, L.A. (1970b) Tentative method of chromatographic analysis for benzo(a)pyrene and benzo(k)fluoranthene in atmospheric particulate matter. Hlth lab. Sci., 7, 60

Sawicki, E., Corey, R.C., Dooley, A.E., Gisclard, J.B., Monkman, J.L., Neligan, R.E. & Ripperton, L.A. (1970c) Tentative method of spectrophotometric analysis for benzo(a)pyrene in atmospheric particulate matter. Hlth lab. Sci., 7, 68

Schaad, R.E. (1970) Chromatographie (karzinogener) polycyclischer aromatischer Kohlenwasserstoffe. Chromat. Rev., 13, 61

Schmit, J.A., Henry, R.A., Williams, R.C. & Dieckman, J.F. (1971) Application of high speed reversed phase liquid chromatography. J. chromat. Sci., 9, 645

Schürch, O. & Winterstein, A. (1935) Über die krebserregende Wirkung aromatischer Kohlenwasserstoffe. Hoppe-Seylers Z. physiol. Chem., 236, 79

Searl, T.D., Cassidy, F.J., King, W.H. & Brown, R.A. (1970) An analytical method for polynuclear aromatic compounds in coke oven effluents by combined use of gas chromatography and ultraviolet absorption spectrometry. Analyt. Chem., 42, 954

Seilern-Aspang, F. & Kratochwil, K. (1962) Induction and differentiation of an epithelial tumour in the newt (Triturus cristatus). J. Embryol. exp. Morphol., 10, 337

Sellakumar, A. & Shubik, P. (1972) Carcinogenicity of 7H-dibenzo(c,g)carbazole in the respiratory tract of hamsters. J. nat. Cancer Inst., 48, 1641

Shabad, L.M. (1968) On the distribution and the fate of the carcinogenic hydrocarbon benz(a)pyrene (3,4-benzpyrene) in the soil. Z. Krebsforsch., 70, 204

Shabad, L.M., Khesina, A.Ya., Linnik, A.B. & Serkovskaya, G.S. (1970) Possible carcinogenic hazards of several tars and of locacorten-tar ointment (spectro-fluorescent investigations and experiments in animals). Int. J. Cancer, 6, 314

Shabad, L.M., Cohan, Y.L., Illnitsky, A.P., Khesina, A. Ya., Shcherbak, N.P. & Smirnov, G.A. (1971) The carcinogenic hydrocarbon benzo(a)pyrene in the soil. J. nat. Cancer Inst., 47, 1179

Shear, M.J. (1938) Studies in carcinogenesis. V. Methyl derivatives of 1,2-benzanthracene. Amer. J. Cancer, 33, 499

Shubik, P. & Hartwell, J.L. (1957) Survey of compounds which have been tested for carcinogenic activity, Washington, D.C., Government Printing Office (Public Health Service Publication No. 149: Supplement 1)

Shubik, P. & Hartwell, J.L. (1969) Survey of compounds which have been tested for carcinogenic activity, Washington, D.C., Government Printing Office (Public Health Service Publication No. 149: Supplement 2)

Shubik, P., Pietra, G. & Della Porta, G. (1960) Studies of skin carcinogenesis in the Syrian golden hamster. Cancer Res., 20, 100

Siddiqui, I. & Wagner, K.H. (1972) Eine universale Methode zur Bestimmung von 3,4-Benzpyren und 3,4-Benzfluoranthen ausgewertet an Regenwasser, Sickerwasser und Weizenproben. Chemosphere, 1, 83

Sims, P. (1967) The metabolism of benzo(a)pyrene by rat-liver homogenates. Biochem. Pharmacol., 16, 613

Sims, P. (1970a) The metabolism of some aromatic hydrocarbons by mouse embryo cell cultures. Biochem. Pharmacol., 19, 285

Sims, P. (1970b) Qualitative and quantitative studies on the metabolism of aromatic hydrocarbons by rat-liver preparations. Biochem. Pharmacol., 19, 795

Smirnov, G.A. (1970) The study of benz(a)pyrene content in soil and vegetation in the airfield region. Vop. Onkol., 16, 83

Smith, C.G., Nau, C.A. & Lawrence, C H. (1968) Separation and identification of polycyclic hydrocarbons in rubber dust. Amer. industr. Hyg. Ass. J., 29, 242

Stanley, T.W., Morgan, M.J. & Meeker, J.E. (1967) Thin-layer chromatographic separation and spectrophotometric determination of benzo(a)pyrene in organic extracts of airborne particles. Analyt. Chem., 39, 1327

Stedman, R.L., Miller, R.L., Lakritz, L. & Chamberlain, W.J. (1968) Methods for concentrating polynuclear aromatic hydrocarbons in cigarette smoke condensate. Chem. and Ind., 394

Stefanescu, A. & Stanescu, L. (1968) Der Gefährdungsgrad unter Einwirkung der aromatischen polynuklearen Kohlenwasserstoffe beim Fabrikationsprozess von Russ. II. Die Gefährdung durch einige krebserzeugende Kohlenwasserstoffe und ihre Bestimmung in der Luft. Z. ges. Hyg., 14, 599

Stocks, P., Commins, B.T. & Aubrey, K.V. (1961) A study of polycyclic hydrocarbons and trace elements in smoke in Merseyside and other northern localities. Int. J. air wat. Pollut., 4, 141

Strömberg, L.E. & Widmark, G. (1970a) Qualitative determination of polyaromatic hydrocarbons in the air near gasworks retorts. J. Chromat., 47, 27

Strömberg, L.E. & Widmark, G. (1970b) Quantitative determination of 3,4-benzopyrene in the air near gas-works retorts. *J. Chromat.*, **49**, 334

Sula, J.P. (1963) The carcinogen 3,4-benzpyrene in the living environment and human organism. *Neoplasma (Bratisl.)*, **10**, 571

Surgeon General's Report (1964) *Smoking and health*, Washington, D.C., Government Printing Office (Public Health Service Publication No. 1103)

Thompson, J.I. & Co. (1971) *Survey of compounds which have been tested for carcinogenic activity*, Washington, D.C., Government Printing Office (Public Health Service Publication No. 149: 1968-1969)

Thorsteinsson, T. (1969) Polycyclic hydrocarbons in commercially and home-smoked food in Iceland. *Cancer*, **23**, 455

Toth, B. & Shubik, P. (1967) Carcinogenesis in AKR mice injected at birth with benzo(a)pyrene and dimethylnitrosamine. *Cancer Res.*, **27**, 43

Tóth, L. (1971) Polyzyklische Kohlenwasserstoffe in geräuchertem Schinken und Bauchspeck. *Fleischwirtschaft*, **7**, 1069

Tracor/Jitco (1973a) *Survey of compounds which have been tested for carcinogenic activity*, Washington, D.C., Government Printing Office (Public Health Service Publication No. 149: 1961-1967) (in press)

Tracor/Jitco (1973b) *Survey of compounds which have been tested for carcinogenic activity*, Washington, D.C., Government Printing Office (Public Health Service Publication No. 149: 1970-1971) (in press)

Tye, R., Horton, A.W. & Rapien, I. (1966) Benzo(a)pyrene and other aromatic hydrocarbons extractable from bituminous coal. *Amer. industr. Hyg. Ass. J.*, **27**, 25

Van Duuren, B.L. (1958) Identification of some polynuclear aromatic hydrocarbons in cigarette smoke condensate. *J. nat. Cancer Inst.*, **21**, 1

Vollmann, H., Becker, H., Corell, M. & Streeck, H. (1937) Beiträge zur Kenntnis des Pyrens und seiner Derivate. *Liebigs Ann. Chem.*, **531**, 1

von Lehmden, D.J., Hangebrauck, R.P. & Meeker, J.E. (1965) Polynuclear hydrocarbon emissions from selected industrial processes. J. air Pollut. Control Ass., 15, 306

Wallcave, L., Garcia, H., Feldman, R., Lijinsky, W. & Shubik, P. (1971) Skin tumorigenesis in mice by petroleum asphalts and coal-tar pitches of known polynuclear aromatic hydrocarbon content. Toxicol. appl. Pharmacol., 18, 41

Waller, R.E. & Commins, B.T. (1967) Studies of the smoke and polycyclic aromatic hydrocarbon content of the air in large urban areas. Environ. Res., 1, 295

Wattenberg, L.W. & Leong, J.L. (1970) Inhibition of the carcinogenic action of benzo(a)pyrene by flavones. Cancer Res., 30, 1922

Wilk, M. & Schwab. H. (1968) Zum Transportphänomen und Wirkungsmechanismus des 3,4-Benzpyrens in der Zelle. Z. Naturforsch., 23B, 431

Wynder, E.L. & Hoffmann, D. (1959) A study of tobacco carcinogenesis. VII. The role of higher polycyclic hydrocarbons. Cancer, 12, 1079

Wynder, E.L. & Hoffmann, D. (1967) Tobacco and tobacco smoke. Studies in experimental carcinogenesis. London, New York, Academic Press

Wynder, E.L., Fritz, L. & Furthe, N. (1957) Effect of concentration of benzopyrene in skin carcinogenesis. J. nat. Cancer Inst., 19, 361

Yanisheva, N.Ya. (1971) The substantiation of the maximum permissible concentration of benz(a)pyrene in the atmosphere of settlements. Gig. i Sanit., 37, 87

Zdrazil, J. & Picha, F. (1966) The occurrence of the carcinogenic compounds 3,4-benzpyrene and arsenic in the soil. Neoplasma, 13, 49

BENZO(e)PYRENE*

1. Chemical and Physical Data

1.1 Synonyms

Chem. Abstr. No.: 192-97-2

4,5-Benzopyrene; 1,2-Benzopyrene; B(e)P

1.2 Chemical formula and molecular weight

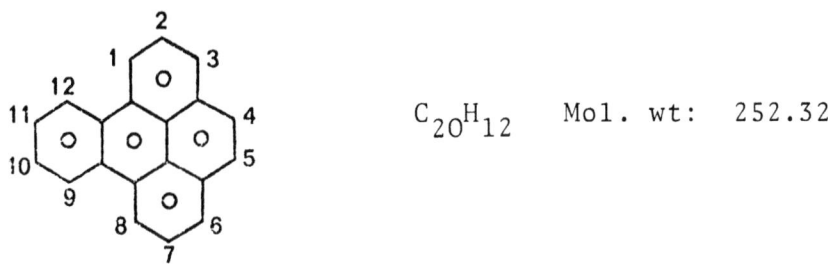

$C_{20}H_{12}$ Mol. wt: 252.32

1.3 Chemical and physical properties of the pure substance

(a) Description: Colourless prisms or plates from alcohol or benzene. General description in Beilsteins handbook, and in Clar (1964).

(b) Boiling-point: 492°C

(c) Melting-point: 178-179°C

(d) Absorption spectroscopy: The ultra-violet absorption spectrum was described in Perkampus et al. (1968), in heptane; by Clar (1964), in ethanol; by Jung & Morand (1963) and Sawicki et al. (1960), in pentane; by Badger et al. (1965); and by Dannenberg & Sonnenbichler (1965), in a DNA solution. The infra-red

---

* Considered by the Working Group in Lyon, December 1972.

absorption spectrum is given in the API Research Project 44 (1960). The fluorescence spectrum is described by Jung & Morand (1963), Sawicki et al. (1960), Van Duuren (1960) and Sawicki (1969), who also discussed the influence of other factors. Data on quasi linear fluorescence and low-temperature fluorescence are given by Dikun (1967), Fedoseeva & Khesina (1968), Hood & Winefordner (1968) and Personov & Solodunov (1968). The nuclear magnetic resonance spectrum is described by Bartle et al. (1969), Cobb & Memory (1967) and Kuthan (1968); and the electron spin resonance spectrum was measured by Griffith & Poole (1969) and by Cooper et al. (1970).

(e) <u>Identity and purity test</u>: Benzo(e)pyrene (B(e)P) forms a picrate with a melting-point of 229-230°C (red needles).

(f) <u>Solubility and/or volatility</u>: 2.9×10^{-8} mol/l dissolve in water at 25°C (Barone et al., 1967). The same paper also contains data on the solubility in water with polymethacrylic acid. The distribution coefficient in the nitromethane/cyclohexane system is 2.10 (Grimmer, 1966). Hoffmann & Wynder (1962b) found distribution coefficients of 1.68 in the same system and 14.5 in the 4:1 cyclohexane/methanol-water system. The solubility of B(e)P with purines and pyrimidines has also been discussed (Caillet & Pullman, 1968).

(g) <u>Chemical reactivity</u>: The relative electron affinities in the gas phase and in solution were detected by potentiometric titration (Chaudri et al., 1967). 6-Bromobenzo(e)pyrene is formed by tetrachlor-o-quinone with HBr (Wilk & Hoppe, 1969). Kuz'min et al. (1967) investigated the mechanism of the electrophilic protonation, and data on the reactive centre (K-region) are given by Hoffmann (1969) and by Sung (1967).

2. Use and Occurrence

(a) Analytical methods

Several chromatographic procedures for the separation of B(e)P from other substances and for its spectroscopic determination have been published and are extensively reviewed by Sawicki (1964) and by Schaad (1970). They include paper chromatography; column chromatography, used for detection in food (Soos & Cieleszky, 1969) and for detection in air (Gladen, 1972); thin-layer chromatography (Janak & Kubecova, 1968; Soos & Cieleszky, 1969; Hood & Winefordner, 1968), used for detection in air (Matsushita & Suzuki, 1969; Strömberg & Widmark, 1970; Brocco et al., 1970), and for detection in paraffin and waxes (Woggon & Jehle, 1966); gas chromatography (Savino, 1968; Bebris et al., 1971; Bhatia, 1971; Gouw et al., 1970; Brocco et al., 1970), used for detection in shale oil (Lahe & Eisen, 1968), for detection in cigarette smoke (Davis, 1969), and for detection in air (Searl et al., 1970); high-speed liquid-liquid chromatography (Schmit et al., 1971); gel chromatography (Edstrom & Petro, 1968); ultra-violet absorption spectroscopy (Strömberg & Widmark, 1970; Searl et al., 1970; Gladen, 1972); fluorescence spectroscopy (Soos & Cieleszky, 1969; Woggon & Jehle, 1966) or low-temperature fluorescence (Hood & Winefordner, 1968); mass spectroscopy (Strömberg & Widmark, 1970); and an electrophoretic separation method (Rothwell & Whitehead, 1967). References to analytical methods used for detection in various other media such as air, cigarette smoke, food, etc. can be found in the section on "Occurrence".

(b) Occurrence

Exhaust: The amounts of B(e)P present in the exhaust of internal combustion engines were determined with a variety of work loads and fuels and with reference to a number of differing parameters. Automobile engines using gasoline as fuel produced 320 µg/kg of soot under idling conditions (zero load) (Falk et al., 1958), while the average of five sampling periods of normal run exhaust soot amounted to 170 mg/kg of particulate matter (Sawicki et al., 1962). From a gasoline engine operated on a simulated city driving schedule 422 mg/kg of exhaust tar were isolated (Hoffmann & Wynder, 1962a) and about 29 µg/ minute run (Hoffmann & Wynder, 1962b, 1963). On a simulated working schedule with a 1000 kg load 33.6 mg/ 1000 m^3 of exhaust were found (Del Vecchio et al., 1970). The output of eight automobiles was 4.7-31.6 µg/mile (Hangebrauck et al., 1966).

Engines using diesel fuel on full load produced 80 mg/kg of soot (Falk et al., 1958), while under various combustions two-cycle engines produced 1.0-8.7 mg/1000 m^3 of exhaust (Reckner et al., 1965). The output of four trucks was about 48 µg/mile (Hangebrauck et al., 1966).

Engines using liquified petroleum gas, while idling under zero load, produced 2.3 mg/1000 m^3, and at full working load 10.8 mg/1000 m^3 of exhaust (Del Vecchio et al., 1970).

Air: B(e)P concentrations in the air depend on the geographic location, the presence nearby of sources of pollution such as traffic highways or industries, and the season. Usually concentrations of B(e)P were greater in urban than non-urban areas and greater in winter than in summer and during periods of increased smoke in the atmosphere.

Detailed studies of air pollution in various cities in Europe (Bosco et al., 1967; Commins & Waller, 1967; Grimmer, 1966), USA (Colucci & Begeman, 1965; DeMaio & Corn, 1966; Epstein et al., 1966; Sawicki et al., 1962; Stocks et al., 1961; Von Lehmden et al., 1965) and Australia (Cleary, 1963; Cleary & Sullivan, 1965) have been reported. Seasonal variations were recorded, winter values ranging from 2.9-208 µg/1000 m^3 and summer values from 0.01-10 µg/1000 m^3 (Bosco et al., 1967; DeMaio & Corn, 1966; Grimmer, 1966; Sawicki et al., 1962; Von Lehmden et al., 1965; Waller & Commins, 1967).

In London, during a period in which smoke condensation was high (December 1957), a concentration as high as 740 µg B(e)P/1000 m^3 was recorded (Commins & Waller, 1967), but after that winter values did not exceed 37 µg/1000 m^3. In Sydney, samples from four different areas of the town showed concentrations of B(e)P ranging between 2.3 and 6.7 µg/1000 m^3 (Cleary, 1963).

Examination of particulates or extracts in six US cities give the following results: 120-630 µg/g of benzene soluble fraction (Sawicki et al., 1965a), and 180-570 µg/g of organic atmospheric particulate matter (Epstein et al., 1966).

In three German cities concentrations ranged from 124-321 µg/kg of dust (Hettche, 1965); and Grimmer & Hildebrandt (1965a) found 23-66 µg/kg in tunnel dust.

Cigarette smoke: In the smoke condensate of 100 cigarettes, concentrations ranging from 0.2-2 µg have been found (Chakraborty et al., 1971; Kiryu & Kuratsune, 1966; Orris et al., 1958; Scassellati-Sforzolini et al., 1967; Van Duuren, 1958; Wynder & Hoffmann, 1963). Wynder & Hoffmann (1959) found 0.1 mg/kg and Elmenhorst & Grimmer (1968) 1.09 mg/kg in cigarette smoke condensate.

Pyrolysis: B(e)P is formed on pyrolysis of anthracene at $950^{\circ}C$ (Badger et al., 1964), of dicetyl at $800^{\circ}C$ (730 mg/kg) (Lam, 1956a), of carbohydrates, amino acids and fatty acids at $700^{\circ}C$ (0.4-32.6 mg/kg) and at $500^{\circ}C$ (up to 0.06 mg/kg) (Masuda et al., 1967), and of different tobacco constituents at $650^{\circ}C$, $700^{\circ}C$ and $800^{\circ}C$ (Badger et al., 1965; Gilbert & Lindsey, 1957; Lam, 1956b).

Occupational exposure: Kreyberg (1959) isolated concentrations of B(e)P ranging from 100-150 µg/1000 m^3 from the air of two gas works and one electrochemical plant. In gas works retort houses, Lawther et al. (1965) found mean concentrations of 900-2500 µg/1000 m^3, while maximum concentrations of 1000 mg/1000 m^3 were measured. Sawicki et al. (1965b) reported 240 µg/1000 m^3 in air contaminated by coal-tar pitch fumes, up to 4300 mg/1000 m^3 in industrial effluents and 500 mg/1000 m^3 in domestic coal combustion stack effluent. B(e)P is present in all kinds of soot and smoke. Hamm & Toth (1970) detected it in tar and smoke from smoke houses, and Rhee & Bratzler (1968) in wood smoke. In carbon black soot, 20-50 mg/kg have been found (Falk et al., 1958), and an average of 3.1 mg/kg (Fischer, 1970) have been detected in different kinds of soot.

The emission levels of B(e)P from heat generation sources ranged from 92-100 000 µg/10^6 Btu[1] heat input (coal) and 18-490 µg/10^6 Btu heat input (gas). From incineration and open burning (of municipal refuse, automobile tyres, etc.) the emission levels ranged from 0.08-6.5 mg/kg of particulate matter for a municipal incinerator, 49-180 mg/kg of particulate matter for a commercial incinerator, and 4.5-450 mg/kg of particulate matter in open burning (Hangebrauck et al., 1964).

The average values for five sampling periods at a downtown garage were 56 µg/kg of particulate matter, and at a safety lane 80 µg/kg of particulate matter (Sawicki et al., 1962).

In commercial waxes, up to 0.039 mg/kg (Lijinsky, 1960) and 12-48 µg/kg (Howard & Haenni, 1963) were found. Lijinsky et al. (1963) detected 0-0.23 mg/kg in petrolatum, 150-180 mg/kg in creosote and 1850-1880 mg/kg in coal-tar samples; and Wallcave et al. (1971) determined a concentration of 0.03-52 mg/kg in petroleum asphalts and 5400-7000 mg/kg in coal-tar pitches.

Food: In meat or fish the amount of B(e)P present depends on the method of cooking: time of exposure, distance of the heat source and whether or not the melted fat is allowed to drop into the heat source. In smoked fish, concentrations ranged from traces to 1.9 µg/kg (Bailey & Dungal, 1958; Grimmer & Hildebrandt, 1967a;

---

[1] British thermal unit

Howard et al., 1966a), while Masuda & Kuratsune (1971) found up to 29 µg/kg. In gas-broiled fish, 1.2 µg/kg were found (Masuda et al., 1966b). Charcoal-broiled or barbecued meat can contain 1.7-7.5 µg/kg (Malanoski et al., 1968; Lijinsky & Shubik, 1964, 1965; Lijinsky & Ross, 1967), and up to 17.5 µg/kg were found in charcoal-broiled T-bone steak (Lijinsky & Ross, 1967). Home smoked meat in Iceland contained up to 4 µg/kg, and 27 µg/kg if the meat was hung close to the stove (Thorsteinsson, 1969). In gas- or electric-broiled meat, the B(e)P content was 0.1-5.7 µg/kg (Grimmer & Hildebrandt, 1967a; Lijinsky & Ross, 1967).

In smoked ham, up to 5.2 µg/kg were found (Grimmer & Hildebrandt, 1967a; Howard et al., 1966a; Hamm & Toth, 1970); heavy smoking brought the B(e)P content up to 17.9 µg/kg (Toth, 1971). Elmenhorst & Dontenwill (1967) detected B(e)P in the smoke of charcoal-broiled bacon, and it has been found in the smoke of gas- and electric-broiled fish (Masuda et al., 1966b).

In vegetables the following amounts of B(e)P were found: salad, 3.7-14.7 µg/kg; tomatoes, 0.2 µg/kg; spinach, 6.9 µg/kg; and kale, 1.1-19.4 µg/kg (Grimmer & Hildebrandt, 1965c). Washing of kale removed only 10% of the quantity. Hettche (1971) found up to 67.2 µg/kg in kale, and Grimmer & Düvel (1970) up to 4.3 µg/kg in soya bean.

Cereals contain variable amounts of B(e)P, depending on their source; concentrations of 0.3-4.9 µg/kg have been found, and this amount is transferred to the flour and bread (Grimmer & Hildebrandt, 1965b; Fritz, 1968c). In the bread crust the content is somewhat higher, depending on the degree of burning (Fritz, 1968c).

In different kinds of crude vegetable oils, concentrations ranged from 0.6-16.5 µg/kg, and up to 32.7 µg/kg have been found in crude coconut oil (Biernoth & Rost, 1967; Grimmer & Hildebrandt, 1967b). B(e)P has also been detected in refined vegetable oils (Jung & Morand, 1963), where concentrations ranging from 0.4-25 µg/kg have been found (Biernoth & Rost, 1968; Howard et al., 1966b). In coconut fat from smoke-dried copra, up to 44 µg/kg have been detected (Biernoth & Rost, 1968) and in different types of margarine and mayonnaise 0.5-1.2 µg/kg (Fritz, 1968a). The B(e)P content of oil decreased slightly with frying (Fritz, 1968d; Berner & Biernoth, 1969).

In roasted coffee, concentrations of B(e)P ranging from 0.3-7.2 µg/kg (Grimmer & Hildebrandt, 1966; Kuratsune & Hueper, 1960; Fritz, 1968b, 1969) were found, depending on the degree of roasting; as much as 20.5 µg/kg were found in malt coffee (Fritz, 1968b).

Black tea extract contained 1.9-22.3 µg/kg B(e)P (Grimmer & Hildebrandt, 1966). In roasted peanuts, up to 0.4 µg/kg B(e)P were found, the amounts rising with the degree of roasting (Ballschmieter, 1969). In baker's dry yeast, Grimmer & Wilhelm (1969) detected 3.1-55 µg/kg B(e)P, while dietetic yeasts or feed yeasts grown on mineral oil showed a lower content. Only in one out of 15 brands of whisky could 0.03 µg/l B(e)P be detected (Masuda et al., 1966a).

Other material: B(e)P has been found in rubber stoppers and in automobile tyres (Falk et al., 1951; Smith et al., 1968), and in furnace blacks (Falk & Steiner, 1952; Smith et al., 1968) in quantities which do not diminish on processing, aging or wear.

3. Biological Data Relevant to the Evaluation of Carcinogenic Risk to Man

3.1 Carcinogenicity and related studies in animals

(<u>a</u>) Skin application

<u>Mouse</u>: Wynder & Hoffmann (1959) painted a group of 20 Swiss mice thrice weekly with a 0.1% solution of B(e)P in acetone. Among eight animals surviving after 10 months, two papillomas and three carcinomas developed. There were no survivors after 14 months.

In the same studies, benzo(a)pyrene and dibenz(a,h)-anthracene at the same or lower concentrations were more active and produced tumours earlier.

A single application of 1.0 mg B(e)P in acetone to the skin of 20 female Swiss mice induced no tumours in an experiment lasting 64 weeks. When this treatment was followed by repeated paintings with croton resin, two out of 20 animals developed one papilloma each (Van Duuren et al., 1968).

3.2 Other relevant biological data

Qualitative and quantitative studies on the metabolism of B(e)P carried out by Sims (1970) showed that 3-hydroxy and 4,5-dihydro-4,5-dihydroxy-benzo(e)pyrene were formed on incubation with a rat liver homogenate.

3.3 Observations in man

None were available to the Working Group.

4. Comments on Data Reported and Evaluation

4.1 Animal data

The data are confined to two skin painting experiments in mice in which B(e)P evoked a weaker response than either benzo(a)pyrene or dibenz(a,h)anthracene. B(e)P does not appear to be an initiator of skin carcinogenesis in mice. It has not been tested by other routes in the mouse or in other species.

4.2 Human data

No case reports or epidemiological studies on the significance of B(e)P exposure to man are available. However, coal-tar and other materials which are known to be carcinogenic to man may contain B(e)P. The substance has also been detected in other environmental situations. The possible contribution of polycyclic aromatic hydrocarbons from some environmental sources to the overall carcinogenic risk to man is discussed in the preamble.

5. References

API Research Project 44 (1960) Selected Infrared Spectral Data, Vol. VI, No. 2249

Badger, G.M., Donnelly, J.K. & Spotswood, T.M. (1964) The formation of aromatic hydrocarbons at high temperatures. XIII. The pyrolysis of anthracene. Aust. J. Chem., 17, 1147

Badger, G.M., Donnelly, J.K. & Spotswood, T.M. (1965) The formation of aromatic hydrocarbons at high temperatures. XXIV. The pyrolysis of some tobacco constituents. Aust. J. Chem., 18, 1249

Bailey, E.J. & Dungal, N. (1958) Polycyclic hydrocarbons in Icelandic smoked food. Brit. J. Cancer, 12, 348

Ballschmieter, H.M.B. (1969) Über polycyclische aromatische Kohlenwasserstoffe in gerösteten Erdnüssen. Fette, Seifen, Anstrichmittel, 71, 521

Barone, G., Crescenzi, V., Liquori, A.M. & Quadrifoglio, F. (1967) Solubilization of polycyclic aromatic hydrocarbons in poly(methacrylic acid) aqueous solution. J. phys. Chem., 71, 2341

Bartle, K.D., Jones, D.W. & Matthews, R.S. (1969) High-field nuclear magnetic resonance spectra of some carcinogenic polynuclear hydrocarbons. Spectrochim. Acta, 25A, 1603

Bebris, N.K., Kiselev, A.V., Mokeev, B.Y., Nikitin, Y.S., Yashin, Y.I. & Zaizeva, G.E. (1971) Macroporous silica as an adsorbent for molecular chromatography. Chromatographia, 4, 93

Beilsteins Handbuch der Organischen Chemie, 5, III, 2520

Berner, G. & Biernoth, G. (1969) Über den Gehalt erhitzter Öle und Fette an polycyclischen aromatischen Kohlenwasserstoffen. Z. Lebensmitt.-Untersuch., 140, 330

Bhatia, K. (1971) Gas chromatographic determination of polycyclic aromatic hydrocarbons. Analyt. Chem., 43, 609

Biernoth, G. & Rost, H.E. (1967) The occurrence of polycyclic aromatic hydrocarbons in coconut oil and their removal. Chem. and Ind., 2002

Biernoth, G. & Rost, H.E. (1968) Vorkommen polycyclischer aromatischer Kohlenwasserstoffe in Speiseölen und deren Entfernung. Arch. Hyg. (Muenchen), 152, 238

Bosco, G., Barsini, G. & Grella, A. (1967) Nuove indagini sulla presenza di idrocarburi policiclici aromatici nel pulviscolo atmosferico del centro storico della citta di Siena. Arch. environ. Hlth, 14, 285

Brocco, D., Cantuti, V. & Cartoni, G.P. (1970) Determination of polynuclear hydrocarbons in atmospheric dust by a combination of thin-layer and gas chromatography. J. Chromat., 49, 66

Caillet, J. & Pullman, B. (1968) Solubilization of aromatic carcinogens by purines and pyrimidines. In: Pullman, B., ed., Molecular Association in Biology, New York, Academic Press, p. 217

Chakraborty, B.B., Kilburn, K.D. & Thornton, R.E. (1971) Reduction in the concentration of aromatic polycyclic hydrocarbons in cigarette smoke. Chem. and Ind., 672

Chaudri, J., Grodzinski, J.J. & Szwarc, M. (1967) Electron affinities of aromatic hydrocarbons in the gas phase and in solution. J. phys. Chem., 71, 3063

Clar, E. (1964) Polycyclic Hydrocarbons, Vol. 2, London, New York, Academic Press; Berlin, Göttingen, Heidelberg, Springer-Verlag, pp. 127, 129

Cleary, G.J. (1963) Measurement of polycyclic aromatic hydrocarbons in the air of Sydney using very long alumina columns for separation. Int. J. air wat. Pollut., 7, 753

Cleary, G.J. & Sullivan, J.L. (1965) Pollution by polycyclic aromatic hydrocarbons in the city of Sydney. Med. J. Aust., 1, 758

Cobb, T.B. & Memory, J.D. (1967) High resolution NMR spectra of polycyclic hydrocarbons. II. Pentacyclic compounds. J. Chem. Phys., 47, 2020

Colucci, J.M. & Begeman, C.R. (1965) The automotive contribution to air-borne polynuclear aromatic hydrocarbons in Detroit. J. air Pollut. Control Ass., 15, 113

Commins, B.T. & Waller, R.E. (1967) Observations from a ten-year study of pollution at a site in the city of London. Atmos. Environ., 1, 49

Cooper, J.T., Forbes, W.F. & Robinson, J.C. (1970) Organic and biological spectrochemical studies. Electron spin resonance spectra of some polynuclear aromatic hydrocarbon ions. Canad. J. Chem., 48, 1942

Dannenberg, H. & Sonnenbichler, J. (1965) Untersuchungen zur Wechselwirkung zwischen aromatischen Kohlenwasserstoffen und Aminen mit Desoxyribonucleinsäure. Z. Krebsforsch., 67, 127

Davis, H.J. (1969) Gas-chromatographic display of the polycyclic aromatic hydrocarbon fraction of cigarette smoke. Talanta, 16, 621

Del Vecchio, V., Valori, P., Melchiorri, C. & Grella, A. (1970) Polycyclic aromatic hydrocarbons from gasoline-engine and liquefied petroleum gas engine exhaust. Pure appl. Chem., 24, 739

DeMaio, L. & Corn, M. (1966) Polynuclear aromatic hydrocarbons associated with particulates in Pittsburgh air. J. air Pollut. Control Ass., 16, 67

Dikun, P.P. (1967) Detection of polycyclic aromatic hydrocarbons in atmospheric contamination and other materials with quasi linear fluorescence spectra. Zh. Prikl. Spektrosk., 6, 202

Edstrom, T. & Petro, B.A. (1968) Gel permeation chromatographic studies of polynuclear aromatic hydrocarbon materials. J. polymer Sci. C, 21, 171

Elmenhorst, H. & Dontenwill, W. (1967) Nachweis cancerogener Kohlenwasserstoffe im Rauch beim Grillen über Holzkohlenfeuer. Z. Krebsforsch., 70, 157

Elmenhorst, H. & Grimmer, G. (1968) Polycyclische Kohlenwasserstoffe aus Zigarettenrauchkondensat. Eine Methode zur Fraktionierung grosser Mengen für Tierversuche. Z. Krebsforsch., 71, 66

Epstein, S.S., Joshi, S., Andrea, J., Mantel, N., Sawicki, E., Stanley, T. & Tabor, E.C. (1966) Carcinogenicity of organic particulate pollutants in urban air after administration of trace quantities to neonatal mice. Nature (Lond.), 212, 1305

Falk, H.L. & Steiner, P.E. (1952) The identification of aromatic polycyclic hydrocarbons in carbon blacks. Cancer Res., 12, 30

Falk, H.L., Steiner, P.E., Goldfein, S., Breslow, A. & Hykes, R. (1951) Carcinogenic hydrocarbons and related compounds in processed rubber. Cancer Res., 11, 318

Falk, H.L., Kotin, P. & Markul, I. (1958) The disappearance of carcinogens from soot in human lungs. Cancer, 11, 482

Fedoseeva, G.E. & Khesina, A.Y. (1968) Use of quasi linear luminescence spectra for the determination of a series of polycyclic hydrocarbons. Zh. Prikl. Spektrosk., 9, 282

Fischer, R. (1970) Spektrophotometrisches Verfahren zur raschen Beurteilung von Russen auf ihren Gehalt an polycyclischen, aromatischen Kohlenwasserstoffen. Z. analyt. Chem., 249, 110

Fritz, W. (1968a) 3,4-Benzpyren und andere Polyaromaten in Margarine und Mayonnaise. Nahrung, 12, 495

Fritz, W. (1968b) Zur Bildung cancerogener Kohlenwasserstoffe bei der thermischen Behandlung von Lebensmitteln. 2. Das Rösten von Bohnenkaffee und Kaffee-Ersatzstoffen. Nahrung, 12, 799

Fritz, W. (1968c) Zur Bildung cancerogener Kohlenwasserstoffe bei der thermischen Behandlung von Lebensmitteln. 3. Das Backen von Brot und Biskuits. Nahrung, 12, 805

Fritz, W. (1968d) Zur Bildung cancerogener Kohlenwasserstoffe bei der thermischen Behandlung von Lebensmitteln. 4. Der Einfluss des Frittierens. Nahrung, 12, 809

Fritz, W. (1969) Zur Lösungsverhalten der Polyaromaten beim Kochen von Kaffee-Ersatzstoffen und Bohnenkaffee. Dtsch. Lebensmitt.-Rdsch., 65, 83

Gilbert, J.A.S. & Lindsey, A.J. (1957) The thermal decomposition of some tobacco constituents. Brit. J. Cancer, 11, 398

Gladen, R. (1972) The determination of carcinogenic polycyclic aromatic hydrocarbons in automobile exhaust gases by column chromatography. Chromatographia, 5, 236

Gouw, T.H., Wittemore, I.M. & Jentoft, R.E. (1970) Versatile short capillary column in gas chromatography. Analyt. Chem., 42, 1394

Griffith, O.F. & Poole, C.P. (1969) Electron spin resonance spectra of negative ions of 1,2-benzopyrene, 1,2,3,4-dibenzanthracene and 3,4-benzophenanthrene. Spectrochim. Acta, 25A, 1463

Grimmer, G. (1966) Cancerogene Kohlenwasserstoffe in der Umgebung des Menschen. Erdöl Kohle-Erdgas-Petrochem., 19, 578

Grimmer, G. & Düvel, D. (1970) Untersuchungen zur endogenen Bildung von polycyclischen Kohlenwasserstoffen in höheren Pflanzen. 8. Cancerogene Kohlenwasserstoffe in der Umgebung des Menschen. Z. Naturforsch., 25B, 1171

Grimmer, G. & Hildebrandt, A. (1965a) Kohlenwasserstoffe in der Umgebung des Menschen. I. Eine Methode zur simultanen Bestimmung von dreizehn polycyclischen Kohlenwasserstoffen. J. Chromat., 20, 89

Grimmer, G. & Hildebrandt, A. (1965b) Kohlenwasserstoffe in der Umgebung des Menschen. II. Der Gehalt polycyclischer Kohlenwasserstoffe in Brotgetreide verschiedener Standorte. Z. Krebsforsch., 67, 272

Grimmer, G. & Hildebrandt, A. (1965c) Kohlenwasserstoffe in der Umgebung des Menschen. III. Der Gehalt polycyclischer Kohlenwasserstoffe in verschiedenen Gemüsesorten und Salaten. Dtsch. Lebensmitt.-Rdsch., 61, 272

Grimmer, G. & Hildebrandt. A. (1966) Der Gehalt polycyclischer Kohlenwasserstoffe in Kaffee und Tee. Dtsch. Lebensmitt.-Rdsch., 62, 19

Grimmer, G. & Hildebrandt, A. (1967a) Kohlenwasserstoffe in der Umgebung des Menschen. V. Der Gehalt polycyclischer Kohlenwasserstoffe in Fleisch und Räucherwaren. Z. Krebsforsch., 69, 223

Grimmer, G. & Hildebrandt, A. (1967b) Content of polycyclic hydrocarbons in crude vegetable oils. Chem. and Ind., 2000

Grimmer, G. & Wilhelm, G. (1969) Der Gehalt von polycyclischen Kohlenwasserstoffen in europäischen Hefen. Dtsch. Lebensmitt.-Rdsch., 65, 229

Hamm, R. & Tóth, L. (1970) Cancerogene Kohlenwasserstoffe in geräucherten Fleischerzeugnissen. Med. u. Ernähr., 11, 25

Hangebrauck, R.P., von Lehmden, D.J. & Meeker, J.E. (1964) Emissions of polynuclear hydrocarbons and other pollutants from heat-generation and incineration processes. J. air Pollut. Control Ass., 14, 267

Hangebrauck, R.P., Lauch, R.P. & Meeker, J.E. (1966) Emissions of polynuclear hydrocarbons from automobiles and trucks. Amer. industr. Hyg. Ass. J., 27, 47

Hettche, H.O. (1965) The measurement of polycyclic aromatics in the atmosphere. Staub (Engl. Transl.), 25, 41

Hettche, H.O. (1971) Plant waxes as collectors of polycyclic aromatics in the air of residential areas. Staub (Engl. Transl.), 31, 34

Hoffmann, D. & Wynder, E.L. (1962a) A study of air pollution carcinogenesis. II. The isolation and identification of polynuclear aromatic hydrocarbons from gasoline engine exhaust condensate. Cancer, 15, 93

Hoffmann, D. & Wynder, E.L. (1962b) Analytical and biological studies on gasoline engine exhaust. Nat. Cancer Inst. Monogr., 9, 91

Hoffmann, D. & Wynder, E.L. (1963) Studies on gasoline engine exhaust. J. air Pollut. Control Ass., 13, 322

Hoffmann, F. (1969) LCAO-MO-SCF Indizes chemischer Reaktions- fähigkeit und krebserregender Eigenschaften polyzyklischer Kohlenwasserstoffe. Theoret. chim. Acta, 15, 393

Hood, L.V. & Winefordner, J.D. (1968) Thin-layer separation and low-temperature luminescence measurement of mixtures of carcinogens. Analyt. chim. Acta, 42, 199

Howard, J.W. & Haenni, E.O. (1963) The extraction and determination of polynuclear hydrocarbons in paraffin waxes. J. Ass. off. agric. Chem., 46, 933

Howard, J.W., Teague, R.T., White, R.H. & Fry, B.E. (1966a) Extraction and estimation of polycyclic aromatic hydrocarbons in smoked foods. I. General method. J. Ass. off. analyt. Chem., 49, 595

Howard, J.W., Turicchi, E.W., White, R.H. & Fazio, T. (1966b) Extraction and estimation of polycyclic aromatic hydrocarbons in vegetable oils. J. Ass. off. analyt. Chem., 49, 1236

Janák, J. & Kubecová, V. (1968) Application of porous ethyl- vinylbenzene polymers to thin-layer chromatography. Separation of aromatic and heterocyclic hydrocarbons and higher phenols on Poropak Q. J. Chromat., 33, 132

Jung, L. & Morand, P. (1963) Présence de pyrène, de benzo- 1,2-pyrène et de benzo-3,4-pyrène dans différentes huiles végétales. C.R. Acad. Sci. (Paris), 257, 1638

Kiryu, S. & Kuratsune, M. (1966) Polycyclic aromatic hydrocarbons in the cigarette tar produced by human smoking. Gann, 57, 317

Kreyberg, L. (1959) 3,4-Benzpyrene in industrial air pollution: some reflexions. Brit. J. Cancer, 13, 618

Kuratsune, M. & Hueper, W.C. (1960) Polycyclic aromatic hydrocarbons in roasted coffee. J. nat. Cancer Inst., 24, 463

Kuthan, J. (1968) Nuclear magnetic resonance spectra and the reactivity of organic compounds. Coll. Cs. Chem. Commun., 33, 1220

Kuz'min, M.G., Ivanov, V.L. & Yakimchenko, O.E. (1967) Use of the fluorescence method for investigations of the mechanism of electrophilic substitution reactions. Khim. Vys. Energ., 1, 443

Lahe, I. & Eisen, O. (1968) Composition of polynuclear aromatic hydrocarbons from heavy fractions of shale oil. Eesti NSV Tead. Akad. Toim., 17, 30

Lam, J. (1956a) Isolation and identification of 3,4-benzpyrene chrysene, and a number of other aromatic hydrocarbons in the pyrolysis products from dicetyl. Acta path. microbiol scand., 39, 198

Lam, J. (1956b) Determination of 3,4-benzpyrene and other aromatic compounds formed by pyrolysis of aliphatic tobacco hydrocarbons. Acta path. microbiol. scand., 39, 207

Lawther, P.J., Commins, B.T. & Waller, R.E. (1965) A study of the concentrations of polycyclic aromatic hydrocarbons in gas works retort houses. Brit. J. industr. Med., 22, 13

Lijinsky, W. (1960) Separation of polycyclic aromatic hydrocarbons in complex mixtures. Analyt. Chem., 32, 684

Lijinsky, W. & Ross, A.E. (1967) Production of carcinogenic polynuclear hydrocarbons in the cooking of food. Food cosmet. Toxicol., 5, 343

Lijinsky, W. & Shubik, P. (1964) Benzo(a)pyrene and other polynuclear hydrocarbons in charcoal-broiled meat. Science, 145, 53

Lijinsky, W. & Shubik, P. (1965) Polynuclear hydrocarbon carcinogens in cooked meat and smoked food. Industr. Med. Surg., 34, 152

Lijinsky, W., Domsky, I., Mason, G., Ramahi, H.Y. & Safavi, T. (1963) The chromatographic determination of trace amounts of polynuclear hydrocarbons in petrolatum, mineral oil, and coal-tar. Analyt. Chem., 35, 952

Malanoski, A.J., Greenfield, E.L., Barnes, C.J., Worthington, J.M. & Joe, F.L. (1968) Survey of polycyclic aromatic hydrocarbons in smoked foods. J. Ass. off. analyt. Chem., 51, 114

Masuda, Y. & Kuratsune, M. (1971) Polycyclic aromatic hydrocarbons in smoked fish, "katsuobushi". Gann, 62, 27

Masuda, Y., Mori, K., Hirohata, T. & Kuratsune, M. (1966a) Carcinogenesis in the esophagus. III. Polycyclic aromatic hydrocarbons and phenols in whisky. Gann, 57, 549

Masuda, Y., Mori, K. & Kuratsune, M. (1966b) Polycyclic aromatic hydrocarbons in common Japanese foods. I. Broiled fish, roasted barley, shoyu, and caramel. Gann, 57, 133

Masuda, Y., Mori, K. & Kuratsune, M. (1967) Polycyclic aromatic hydrocarbons formed by pyrolysis of carbohydrates, amino acids and fatty acids. Gann, 58, 69

Matsushita, H. & Suzuki, Y. (1969) Two-dimensional dual-band thin-layer chromatographic separation of polynuclear hydrocarbons. Bull. Chem. Soc. Japan, 42, 460

Orris, L., Van Duuren, B.L. & Kosak, I.K. (1958) The carcinogenicity for mouse skin and the aromatic hydrocarbon content of cigarette smoke condensates. J. nat. Cancer Inst., 21, 557

Perkampus, H.H., Sandeman, I. & Timmons, C.J., eds. (1968) DMS UV Atlas of Organic Compounds, Vol. IV, Weinheim, Verlag Chemie; London, Butterworths, H 16/2a

Personov, R.I. & Solodnunov, V.V. (1968) Temperature broadening, shift and line shape in quasi-linear spectra of organic molecules in crystalline normal paraffin solution. Fisik. Tverd. Tela, 10, 1848

Reckner, L.R., Scott, W.E. & Biller, W.F. (1965) The composition and odor of diesel exhaust. Proc. amer. petrol. Inst. 45, 133

Rhee, K.S. & Bratzler, L.J. (1968) Polycyclic hydrocarbon composition of wood smoke. J. food Sci., 33, 626

Rothwell, K. & Whitehead, J.K. (1967) A method for the isolation of polycyclic aromatic hydrocarbons from complex hydrocarbon mixtures. Chem. and Ind., 784

Savino, A. (1968) Determinazione per via gas chromatographica degli idrocarburi aromatici policiclici. Riv. ital. Igiene, 28, 56

Sawicki, E. (1964) The separation and analysis of polynuclear aromatic hydrocarbons present in the human environment. I-III. Chemist-Analyst, 53, 24, 56, 88

Sawicki, E. (1969) Fluorescence analysis in air pollution research. Talanta, 16, 1231

Sawicki, E., Hauser, T.R. & Stanley, T.W. (1960) Ultraviolet, visible and fluorescent spectral analysis of polynuclear hydrocarbons. Int. J. air. Pollut., 2, 253

Sawicki, E., Hauser, T.R., Elbert, W.C., Fox, F.T. & Meeker, J.E. (1962) Polynuclear aromatic hydrocarbon composition of the atmosphere in some large American cities. Amer. industr. Hyg. Ass. J., 23, 137

Sawicki, E., McPherson, S.P., Stanley, T.W., Meeker, J.E. & Elbert, W.C. (1965a) Quantitative composition of the urban atmosphere in terms of polynuclear aza heterocyclic compounds and aliphatic and polynuclear aromatic hydrocarbons. Int. J. air wat. Pollut., 9, 515

Sawicki, E., Meeker, J.E. & Morgan, M.J. (1965b) The quantitative composition of air pollution source effluents in terms of aza heterocyclic compounds and polynuclear aromatic hydrocarbons. Int. J. air wat. Pollut., 9, 291

Scassellati-Sforzolini, G., Pascasio, F., Mastrandrea, F. & Savino, A. (1967) Attività cancerigena del fumo di sigaretta. Quantificazione degli idrocarburi aromatici policiclici presenti nell porzione aspirata. Riv. ital. Igiene, 27, 175

Schaad, R. (1970) Chromatographie (karzinogener) polyzyklischer aromatischer Kohlenwasserstoffe. Chromat. Rev., 13, 61

Schmit, J.A., Henry, R.A., Williams, R.C. & Dieckman, J.F. (1971) Applications of high speed reversed-phase liquid chromatography. J. chromat. Sci., 9, 645

Searl, T.D., Cassidy, F.J., King, W.H. & Brown, R.A. (1970) An analytical method for polynuclear aromatic compounds in coke oven effluents by combined use of gas chromatography and ultraviolet absorption spectrometry. Analyt. Chem., 42, 954

Sims, P. (1970) Qualitative and quantitative studies on the metabolism of a series of aromatic hydrocarbons by rat-liver preparations. Biochem. Pharmacol., 19, 795

Smith, C.G., Nau, C.A. & Lawrence, C.H. (1968) Separation and identification of polycyclic hydrocarbons in rubber dust. Amer. industr. Hyg. Ass. J., 29, 242

Soos, K. & Cieleszyk, V. (1969) Qualitative and quantitative investigation of cancerogenic polycyclic hydrocarbons in foods in contacting mineral oil derivatives. Kolor. Ert., 11, 100

Stocks, P., Commins, B.T. & Aubrey, K.V. (1961) A study of polycyclic hydrocarbons and trace elements in smoke in Merseyside and other northern localities. Int. J. air wat. Pollut., 4, 141

Strömberg, L.E. & Widmark, G. (1970) Qualitative determination of polyaromatic hydrocarbons in the air near gas-works retorts. J. Chromat., 47, 27

Sung, S. (1967) Sur l'existence eventuelle d'une correlation plus générale entre le pouvoir cancérogène d'une substance et une de ses propriétées moléculaires. C.R. Acad. Sci. (Paris), Ser. D, 264, 189

Thorsteinsson, T. (1969) Polycyclic hydrocarbons in commercially and home-smoked food in Iceland. Cancer Res., 20, 1538

Tóth, L. (1971) Polyzyklische Kohlenwasserstoffe in geräuchertem Schinken und Bauchspeck. Fleischwirtschaft, 7, 1069

Van Duuren, B.L. (1958) The polynuclear aromatic hydrocarbons in cigarette-smoke condensate. II. J. nat. Cancer Inst., 21, 623

Van Duuren, B.L. (1960) The fluorescence spectra of aromatic hydrocarbons and heterocyclic aromatic compounds. Analyt. Chem., 32, 1436

Van Duuren, B.L., Sivak, A., Langseth, L. & Goldschmidt, B. (1968) Initiators and promoters in tobacco carcinogenesis. J. nat. Cancer Inst., 28, 173

von Lehmden, D.J., Hangebrauck, R.P. & Meeker, J.E. (1965) Polynuclear hydrocarbon emissions from selected industrial processes. J. air Pollut. Control Ass., 15, 306

Wallcave, L., Garcia, H., Feldman, R., Lijinsky, W. & Shubik, P. (1971) Skin tumorigenesis in mice by petroleum asphalts and coal-tar pitches of known polynuclear aromatic hydrocarbon content. Toxicol. appl. Pharmacol., 18, 41

Waller, R.E. & Commins, B.T. (1967) Studies of the smoke and polycyclic aromatic hydrocarbon content of the air in large urban areas. Environ. Res., 1, 295

Wilk, M. & Hoppe, U. (1969) Nucleophile Substitution carcinogener und nichtcarcinogener Kohlenwasserstoffe über Elektronen-Donator-Acceptor Komplexe. Liebigs Ann. Chem., 727, 81

Woggon, H. & Jehle, D. (1966) Zum dünnschichtchromatographischen Nachweis kanzerotener Kohlenwasserstoffe in Paraffinen und Wachsen. Plaste und Kautschuk, 13, 460

Wynder, E.L. & Hoffmann, D. (1959) A study of tobacco carcinogenesis. VII. The role of higher polycyclic hydrocarbons. Cancer, 12, 1079

Wynder, E.L. & Hoffmann, D. (1963) Ein experimenteller Beitrag zur Tabakrauchkanzerogenese. Dtsch. med. Wschr., 88, 623

CHRYSENE*

1. Chemical and Physical Data

1.1 Synonyms

Chem. Abstr. No.: 218-01-9

1,2-Benzophenanthrene; Benz(a)phenanthrene;
1,2,5,6-Dibenzonaphthalene

1.2 Chemical formula and molecular weight

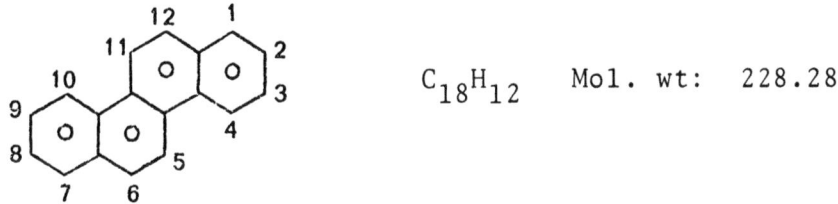

$C_{18}H_{12}$ Mol. wt: 228.28

1.3 Chemical and physical properties of the pure substance

(<u>a</u>) Description: Colourless platelets which show a blue fluorescence. General description in Beilsteins handbook, and in Clar (1964).

(<u>b</u>) Boiling-point: 448°C

(<u>c</u>) Melting-point: 255.8-256.3°C (corr.)

(<u>d</u>) Density: D_4^{20} = 1.274

(<u>e</u>) Absorption spectroscopy: The ultra-violet absorption spectrum is described by Sawicki et al. (1960a, b), in pentane; by Clar (1964), in ethanol; and by Badger et al. (1965). The fluorescence spectrum is given by Van Duuren (1958); by

---

* Considered by the Working Group in Lyon, December 1972.

Schoental & Scott (1949), in petroleum ether; and by Sawicki et al. (1960a,b), in pentane. The infrared absorption spectrum is given in the API Research Project 44 (1960).

(f) <u>Identity and purity test</u>: Chrysene forms crystalline complexes with picric acid (orange-red needles from benzene, melting-point 174-175°C corr.), s-trinitrobenzene (188.5-189.5°C corr.) and 2,4,7-trinitrofluorenone (yellow needles from alcohol, melting point 247.8-249°C).

(g) <u>Solubility and/or volatility</u>: One hundred parts ethanol dissolve 0.097 parts chrysene at 16°C and 0.17 parts at 78°C. One hundred parts toluene dissolve 0.24 parts chrysene at 18°C and 5.39 parts at 100°C. It is sparingly soluble in glacial acetic acid, ether and carbon disulphide and slightly soluble in hot benzene or xylene. Distribution coefficients in the methanol-water/nitromethane system are given by Hoffmann & Wynder (1962a). Chrysene sublimes <u>in vacuo</u>.

(h) <u>Chemical reactivity</u>: Chrysene is first substituted in the 6 position by electrophilic reactions and then yields disubstituted products. 5,6-Chrysoquinone is formed in a boiling solution of chromic acid in glacial acetic acid. Chrysene is oxidized by osmium tetroxide in pyridine to 5,6-dihydro-1,2-dihydroxychrysene (Clar, 1964).

2. Use and Occurrence

(a) Analytical methods

Several chromatographic procedures for the separation of chrysene from other substances and for its spectroscopic determination have been published and are extensively reviewed by Sawicki (1964) and by Schaad (1970). They include paper chromatography; column chromatography, used for detection in air (Sawicki et al., 1970); thin-layer chromatography; gas chromatography, used for detection in soot (Chakraborty & Long, 1967), and for detection in air (Searl et al., 1970); gel chromatography (Edstrom & Petro, 1968); ultra-violet absorption spectroscopy (Sawicki et al., 1970; Searl et al., 1970); and fluorescence spectroscopy. References to analytical methods used for detection in various other media such as air, water, food, etc. can be found in the section on "Occurrence".

(b) Occurrence

Exhaust: Hoffmann & Wynder (1962a,b, 1963) isolated 12 µg chrysene from automobile exhaust gas after a one-minute run, and 175 mg/kg of exhaust tar from gasoline engine exhaust. Two-cycle diesel engines under various conditions produced 3.6-17 µg/m^3 of exhaust (Reckner et al., 1965).

Air: Detailed studies of air pollution in various cities in Europe, USA and Australia showed that in general concentrations depended on the geographic location, the presence of nearby sources of pollution such as traffic highways or industries, and the season. Usually, concentrations were greater in winter than in summer. In Siena, Pittsburgh and Bochum, seasonal variations were recorded; summer values ranged from

2.5-3.6 µg/1000 m^3 (Bosco et al., 1967; DeMaio & Corn, 1966) and winter values from 20-361 µg/1000 m^3 (Bosco et al., 1967; DeMaio & Corn, 1966; Grimmer, 1966). In Sydney and Cincinnati concentrations of 1.8-13.3 µg/1000 m^3 (Cleary, 1963; Conlee et al., 1967), depending on the traffic situation, were found. Examination of particulates or extracts give the following results: 150-490 µg/g of organic atmospheric particulate matter in six American cities (Epstein et al., 1966); 200-533 µg/kg in three German cities (Hettche, 1965); 5.4 (winter value) - 23.3 µg/g (summer value) in Sydney (Cleary & Sullivan, 1965); 22-64 µg/kg in road dust near a highway (Borneff & Kunte, 1965); and 42.6-119 µg/g in dust samples from an automobile tunnel (Grimmer & Hildebrandt, 1965a).

Cigarette smoke: In the smoke condensate of 100 cigarettes, concentrations ranging from 0.06-6.0 µg were found (Cook, 1961; Kiryu & Kuratsune, 1966; Van Duuren, 1958; Wynder & Hoffmann, 1963), and in smoke condensate 1.5-2 µg/kg (Wynder & Hoffmann, 1959) and 5.7 µg/g (Elmenhorst & Grimmer, 1968).

Pyrolysis: Chrysene is formed on pyrolysis of dicetyl at 800°C (0.17 mg/kg) (Lam, 1956a), of aliphatic hydrocarbons in tobacco at 800°C (0.4 mg/kg) and at 700°C (0.086 mg/kg) (Lam, 1956b) and of carbohydrates, amino acids and fatty acids at 700°C (up to 91 mg/kg) and at 500°C (up to 0.16 mg/kg) but none at 300°C (Masuda et al., 1967).

Occupational exposure: Chrysene has been determined by Sawicki et al. (1965) in the effluents of two industrial sources (1600 mg/1000 m^3). It has been found in different kinds of soot and smoke, e.g., in carbon black soot (45-200 µg/m^3) (Stefanescu & Stanescu, 1968), in wood smoke (Rhee & Bratzler, 1968), and in soot from pre-mixed acetylene-oxygen flames (Long & Tompkins, 1967). In addition, chrysene occurs in the aromatic fraction of a clarified oil (Dietz et al., 1956); in commercial solvents (Lijinsky & Raha, 1961), and waxes (2 µg/kg) (Howard & Haenni, 1963); in tar oil for impregnation of timber (Kadlec et al., 1962); in gas works tar (Kennaway, 1924); in paraffin wax (Lijinsky et al., 1961); in petrolatum (up to 0.44 mg/kg), creosote (up to 1340 mg/kg) and coal-tar (up to 2860 mg/kg) (Lijinsky et al., 1963); in benzene extracts of Yubari coal (Ouchi & Imuta, 1963); in cracked petroleum residuum and extracts of bituminous coal (Tye et al., 1966a,b); in extracts from the Posidonomya shales (Heller, 1967); and in petroleum asphalts (0.4-34 mg/kg) and coal-tar pitch (up to 10 000 mg/kg) (Wallcave et al., 1971).

<u>Soil and water</u>: Fritz & Engst (1971) found 15 µg/kg in sand samples and up to 600 000 µg/kg in soil polluted by coal-tar pitch, and Blumer (1961) detected chrysene in rural soil.

Chrysene has been reported to be present in surface water at concentrations of 11.8-38.2 µg/m^3, measured at different times (Borneff & Kunte, 1964). It occurred in all water samples of the tributaries of Lake Constance, but quantitative determination was possible in only one case (1.6 mg/kg) (Borneff & Kunte, 1965).

Food: In meat or fish the amount of chrysene present depends on the method of cooking: time of exposure, distance of the heat source and whether or not the melted fat is allowed to drop into the heat source. In broiled meat and sausages, concentrations ranged from 0.5-2.6 µg/kg (Grimmer & Hildebrandt, 1967a; Malanoski et al., 1968). In ham, 0.5-2.6 µg/kg were found (Malanoski et al., 1968), while heavy smoking brought the chrysene content up to 21.2 µg/kg (Tóth, 1971). In charcoal-broiled or barbecued meat, concentrations ranging from 0.6-25.4 µg/kg (Lijinsky & Ross, 1967; Malanoski et al., 1968) were found. In gas-broiled fish, up to 4.3 µg/kg were detected (Masuda et al., 1966b); and in smoked fish, concentrations ranged from 0.3-173 µg/kg (Grimmer & Hildebrandt, 1967a; Lijinsky & Shubik, 1965a; Masuda & Kuratsune, 1971). In the smoke of charcoal-broiled bacon (Elmenhorst & Dontenwill, 1967) and of gas- and electric-broiled fish (Masuda et al., 1966b), chrysene could be detected; and Lijinsky & Shubik (1965b) found 0-6 µg/kg in liquid smoke.

In vegetables, the following amounts of chrysene were found: salad, 5.7-26.5 µg/kg; spinach, 28.0 µg/kg; tomatoes, 0.5 µg/kg; and kale, 58.5-395 µg/kg (Grimmer & Hildebrandt, 1965c; Hettche, 1971).

Cereals (wheat, barley and rye) were contaminated to variable degrees (0.8-14.5 µg/kg) with chrysene, depending on their source (Grimmer & Hildebrandt, 1965b).

In different kinds of refined vegetable oils, mean values were between 0.5-16.4 µg/kg (Grimmer & Hildebrandt, 1967b); and up to 20 µg/l in pressed or rectified olive oil (Ciusa et al., 1968), up to 129 µg/kg in crude coconut oil (Biernoth & Rost, 1967; Grimmer & Hildebrandt, 1967b) and up to 200 µg/kg in crude coconut fat (Biernoth & Rost, 1968) have been found. The chrysene content of oils was reduced slightly by frying (Berner & Biernoth, 1969).

In roasted coffee or soluble coffee powder, concentrations ranging from 0.6-19.1 µg/kg (Grimmer & Hildebrandt, 1966; Kuratsune & Hueper, 1960; Fritz, 1969) have been found; and in black tea extracts, 4.6-6.3 µg/kg were detected (Grimmer & Hildebrandt, 1966). In peanuts roasted to two different degrees, 0.01-0.71 µg/kg were found (Ballschmieter, 1969). In baker's dry yeast 42-203 µg/kg were detected, while dietetic yeast or feed yeast grown on mineral oil showed a lower content (Grimmer & Wilhelm, 1969). Masuda et al. (1966a) found chrysene in two kinds of whisky in concentrations of 0.04-0.06 µg/l.

Other material: Falk et al. (1951) identified chrysene in extracts of rubber stoppers and automobile tyres.

3. Biological Data Relevant to the Evaluation of Carcinogenic Risk to Man

3.1 Carcinogenicity and related studies in animals

(a) Skin application

Mouse: In an old experiment, mice were painted twice weekly with different samples of chrysene as a 0.3% solution in benzene for over 440 days. A sample of chrysene of doubtful purity produced two papillomas among 50 mice (30 of which were alive at six months);

another sample produced one papilloma and one epithelioma among 100 mice (74 of which were alive at six months); whereas a sample of synthetic chrysene did not induce tumours among 20 mice (11 alive at six months). A 0.3% solution in mouse fat or a 7.5% solution in oleic acid did not produce tumours among 120 mice (Barry et al., 1935). Another study with an unspecified concentration of "pure" chrysene in benzene did not produce tumours among 50 mice, 11 of which were alive after 276 days (Schürch & Winterstein, 1935). In another experiment, in which synthetic chrysene was painted as a 0.3% concentration in benzene twice weekly, five of 20 mice lived longer than 440 days and one developed a papilloma at 711 days (Bachmann et al., 1937). Riegel et al. (1951) induced one epithelioma among 16 CF1 mice surviving after 31 weeks of biweekly painting with a 0.2% solution in acetone.

In a more recent experiment, among 20 female Swiss mice painted thrice weekly with a 1% solution of chrysene in acetone, papillomas appeared in nine animals and carcinomas in eight, the first tumour being observed after eight months. There was an obvious shortening of the lifespan (Wynder & Hoffmann, 1959).

A single application of 1 mg of chrysene in acetone did not produce tumours within 63 weeks. The same treatment initiated carcinogenesis when it was followed by repeated painting with croton resin; it then induced papillomas in 16 mice out of 20, as well as two carcinomas (Van Duuren et al., 1966)

(b) Subcutaneous and/or intramuscular administration

Mouse: One s.c. injection of 2 mg purified chrysene did not produce sarcomas among 50 mice observed for 45 weeks (Bottomley & Twort, 1934). Similarly, two subcutaneous implantations of 10 mg each to 30 mice gave negative results (Shear & Leiter, 1941). Steiner & Falk (1951) obtained four sarcomas among 50 C57BL mice (39 of which survived after four months) injected s.c. with 5 mg chrysene in tricapryline; the average induction time was 401 days, and the experiments terminated at 22 months. Steiner (1955) injected 5 mg chrysene in tricapryline to 40 or 50 C57BL mice; 22 mice were alive at 150 days, and five developed sarcomas. The average induction time was 271 days and the experiment terminated between 22 and 28 months. In another experiment on the same strain of mice, 2/20 animals developed tumours 60-80 weeks after 10 injections of 1 mg chrysene in arachis oil (no tumours appeared in controls given the solvent alone) (Boyland & Sims, 1967).

Rat: Barry & Cook (1934) gave repeated injections of chrysene in lard at doses of 2-3 mg and observed four tumours among 10 rats, whereas 2/10 controls given the solvent only also developed sarcomas. Bi-weekly injections of a 0.05% aqueous colloidal solution of purified chrysene did not produce tumours among 10 rats, four of which were alive at 18 months (Boyland & Burrows, 1935).

(c) Intraperitoneal administration

Mouse: In an experiment lasting 50 weeks, no tumours appeared among 50 mice given an injection of 2 mg chrysene in lard (Bottomly & Twort, 1934).

3.2 Other relevant biological data

Quantitative experiments (Sims, 1970) using labelled chrysene showed that four phenols were formed by rat liver homogenates: the main phenol is probably 1-hydroxy-chrysene, and two of the dihydro-dihydroxy compounds are probably 1,2-dihydro-1,2-dihydroxychrysene and 3,4-dihydro-3,4-dihydroxy-chrysene.

3.3 Observations in man

None were available to the Working Group.

4. Comments on Data Reported and Evaluation

4.1 Animal data

Chrysene has produced skin tumours in mice following repeated paintings in the only study in which a concentration as high as 1% in acetone was used. It is also an initiator of skin carcinogenesis in mice, whereas a single painting with 1 mg chrysene with no further treatment did not induce tumours.

High doses (2-20 mg) given by s.c. injection to mice produced a low incidence of tumours with a long induction time.

It has not been adequately tested by other routes or in other species.

4.2 Human data

No case reports or epidemiological studies on the significance of chrysene exposure to man are available. However, coal-tar and other materials which are known to be carcinogenic to man may contain chrysene. The substance has also been detected in other environmental situations. The possible contribution of polycyclic aromatic hydrocarbons from some environmental sources to the overall carcinogenic risk to man is discussed in the preamble.

5. References

API Research Project 44 (1960) Selected Infrared Spectral Data, Vol. VI, No. 2241

Bachmann, W.E., Cook, J.W., Dansi, A., de Worms, C.G.M., Haslewood, G.A.D., Hewett, C.L. & Robinson, A.M. (1937) The production of cancer by pure hydrocarbons. IV. Proc. roy. Soc. London B, 123, 343

Badger, G.M., Donnelly, J.K. & Spotswood, T.M. (1965) The formation of aromatic hydrocarbons at high temperatures. XXIV. The pyrolysis of some tobacco constituents. Aust. J. Chem., 18, 1249

Ballschmieter, H.M.B. (1969) Über polycyclische aromatische Kohlenwasserstoffe in gerösteten Erdnüssen. Fette, Seifen, Anstrichmittel, 71, 521

Barry, G. & Cook, J.W. (1934) A comparison of the action of some polycyclic aromatic hydrocarbons in producing tumours of connective tissue. Amer. J. Cancer, 20, 58

Barry, G., Cook, J.W., Haslewood, G.A.D., Hewett, C.L., Hieger, I. & Kennaway, E.L. (1935) The production of cancer by pure hydrocarbons. III. Proc. roy. Soc. London B, 117, 318

Beilsteins Handbuch der Organischen Chemie, 5, 718; 5, 1, 355; 5, II, 629; 5, III, 2380

Berner, G. & Biernoth, G. (1969) Über den Gehalt erhitzter Öle und Fette an polycyclischen aromatischen Kohlenwasserstoffen. Z. Lebensmitt.-Untersuch., 140, 330

Biernoth, G. & Rost, H.E. (1967) The occurrence of polycyclic aromatic hydrocarbons in coconut oil and their removal. Chem. and Ind., 2002

Biernoth, G. & Rost, H.E. (1968) Vorkommen polycyclischer aromatischer Kohlenwasserstoffe in Speiseölen und deren Entfernung. Arch. Hyg. (Muenchen), 152, 238

Blumer, M. (1961) Benzpyrenes in soil. Science, 134, 474

Borneff, J. & Kunte, H. (1964) Kanzerogene Substanzen in Wasser und Boden. XVI. Nachweis von polyzyklischen Aromaten in Wasserproben durch direkte Extraction. Arch. Hyg. (Muenchen), 148, 585

Borneff, J. & Kunte, H. (1965) Kanzerogene Substanzen in Wasser und Boden. XVII. Uber die Herkunft und Bewertung der polyzyklischen aromatischen Kohlenwasserstoffe in Wasser. Arch. Hyg. (Muenchen), 149, 226

Bosco, G., Barsini, G. & Grella, A. (1967) Nuove indagini sulla presenza di idrocarburi policiclici aromatici nel pulviscolo atmosferico del centro storico della citta di Siena. Arch. environ. Hlth, 14, 285

Bottomley, A.C. & Twort, C.C. (1934) The carcinogenicity of chrysene and oleic acid. Amer. J. Cancer, 21, 781

Boyland, E. & Burrows, H. (1935) The experimental production of sarcoma in rats and mice by a colloidal aqueous solution of 1,2,5,6-dibenzanthracene. J. Path. Bact., 41, 231

Boyland, E. & Sims, P. (1967) The carcinogenic activities in mice of compounds related to benz(a)anthracene. Int. J. Cancer, 2, 500

Chakraborty, B.B. & Long, R. (1967) Gas chromatographic analysis of polycyclic aromatic hydrocarbons in soot samples. Environ. Sci. Technol., 1, 828

Ciusa, W., D'Arrigo, V., Maini, F. & Penna, N. (1968) Sul contenuto in idrocarburi policiclici aromatici degli oli di oliva. Riv. ital. Sost. grasse, 45, 175

Clar, E. (1964) Polycyclic Hydrocarbons, Vol. 1, London, New York, Academic Press; Berlin, Göttingen, Heidelberg, Springer-Verlag, p. 243

Cleary, G.J. (1963) Measurement of polycyclic aromatic hydrocarbons in the air of Sydney using very long alumina columns for separation. Int. J. air wat. Pollut., 7, 753

Cleary, G.J. & Sullivan, J.L. (1965) Pollution by polycyclic aromatic hydrocarbons in the city of Sydney. Med. J. Aust., 1, 758

Conlee, C.J., Kenline, P.A., Cummins, R.L. & Konopinski, V.J. (1967) Motor vehicle exhaust at three selected sites. Arch. environ. Hlth, 14, 429

Cook, J.W. (1961) Tobacco Smoke and Lung Cancer. The Royal Institute of Chemistry Lecture Series, No. 5

DeMaio, L. & Corn, M. (1966). Polynuclear aromatic hydrocarbons associated with particulates in Pittsburgh air. J. air Pollut. Control Ass., 16, 67

Dietz, W.A., Dudenbostal, B.F. & Priestley, W. (1956) Analysis of high boiling petroleum fractions by ultra violet spectrometry. Amer. chem. Soc., Div. petrol. Chem. Preprints, 1, 117

Edstrom, T. & Petro, B.A. (1968) Gel permeation chromatographic studies of polynuclear aromatic hydrocarbon material. J. polymer Sci. C, 21, 171

Elmenhorst, H. & Dontenwill, W. (1967) Nachweis cancerogener Kohlenwasserstoffe im Rauch beim Grillen über Holzhohlenfeuer. Z. Krebsforsch., 70, 157

Elmenhorst, H. & Grimmer, G. (1968) Polycyclische Kohlenwasserstoffe aus Zigarettenrauchkondensat. Eine Methode zur Fraktionierung grosser Mengen für Tierversuche. Z. Krebsforsch., 71, 60

Epstein, S.S., Joshi, S., Andrea, J., Mantel, N., Sawicki, E., Stanley, T. & Tabor, E.C. (1966) Carcinogenicity of organic particulate pollutants in urban air after administration of trace quantities to neonatal mice. Nature (Lond.), 212, 1305

Falk, H.L., Steiner, P.E., Goldfein, S., Breslow, A. & Hykes, R. (1951) Carcinogenic hydrocarbons and related compounds in processed rubber. Cancer Res., 11, 318

Fritz, W. (1969) Zur Lösungsverhalten der Polyaromaten beim Kochen von Kaffee-Ersatzstoffen und Bohnenkaffee. Dtsch. Lebensmitt.-Rdsch., 65, 83

Fritz, W. & Engst, R. (1971) Zur umweltbedington Kontamination von Lebensmitteln mit krebserzeugenden Kohlenwasserstoffen. Z. ges. Hyg., 17, 271

Grimmer, G. (1966) Cancerogene Kohlenwasserstoffe in der Umgebung des Menschen. Erdöl Kohle-Erdgas-Petrochem., 19, 578

Grimmer, G. & Hildebrandt, A. (1965a) Kohlenwasserstoffe in der Umgebung des Menschen. I. Eine Methode zur simultanen Bestimmung von dreizehn polycyclischen Kohlenwasserstoffen. J. Chromat., 20, 89

Grimmer, G. & Hildebrandt, A. (1965b) Kohlenwasserstoffe in der Umgebung des Menschen. II. Der Gehalt polycyclischer Kohlenwasserstoffe in Brotgetreide verschiedener Standorte. Z. Krebsforsch., 67, 272

Grimmer, G. & Hildebrandt, A. (1965c) Kohlenwasserstoffe in der Umgebung des Menschen. III. Der Gehalt polycyclischer Kohlenwasserstoffe in verschiedenen Gemüsesorten und Salaten. Dtsch. Lebensmitt.-Rdsch., 61, 272

Grimmer, G. & Hildebrandt, A. (1966) Der Gehalt polycyclischer Kohlenwasserstoffe in Kaffee und Tee. Dtsch. Lebensmitt.-Rdsch., 62, 19

Grimmer, G. & Hildebrandt, A. (1967a) Kohlenwasserstoffe in der Umgebung des Menschen. V. Der Gehalt polycyclischer Kohlenwasserstoffe in Fleisch und Räucherwaren. Z. Krebsforsch., 69, 223

Grimmer, G. & Hildebrandt, A. (1967b) Content of polycyclic hydrocarbons in crude vegetable oils. Chem. and Ind., 2000

Grimmer, G. & Wilhelm, G. (1969) Der Gehalt von polycyclischen Kohlenwasserstoffen in europäischen Hefen. Dtsch. Lebensmitt.-Rdsch., 65, 229

Heller, V.W. (1967) Hydrocarbons and fats in the distillates and extracts from the Posidonomya shales of Swabia. Erdöl Kohle-Erdgas-Petrochem., 20, 709

Hettche, H.O. (1965) The measurement of polycyclic aromatics in the atmosphere. Staub (Engl. Transl.), 25, 41

Hettche, H.O. (1971) Plant waxes as collectors of polycyclic aromatics in the air of residential areas. Staub (Engl. Transl.), 31, 34

Hoffmann, D. & Wynder, E.L. (1962a) Analytical and biological studies on gasoline engine exhaust. Nat. Cancer Inst. Monogr., 9, 91

Hoffmann, D. & Wynder, E.L. (1962b) A study of air pollution carcinogenesis. II. The isolation and identification of polynuclear aromatic hydrocarbons from gasoline engine exhaust condensate. Cancer, 15, 93

Hoffmann, D. & Wynder, E.L. (1963) Studies on gasoline engine exhaust. J. air Pollut. Control Ass., 13, 322

Howard, J.W. & Haenni, E.O. (1963) The extraction and determination of polynuclear hydrocarbons in paraffin waxes. J. Ass. off. agric. Chem., 46, 933

Kadlec, K., Hanslian, L. & Barborik, M. (1962) Occupational carcinoma of the skin in work with tar oils. Pracov. Lek., 14, 170

Kennaway, E.L. (1924) On the cancer-producing factor in tar. Brit. med. J., i, 564

Kiryu, S. & Kuratsune, M. (1966) Polycyclic aromatic hydrocarbons in the cigarette tar produced by human smoking. Gann, 57, 317

Kuratsune, M. & Hueper, W.C. (1960) Polycyclic aromatic hydrocarbons in roasted coffee. J. nat. Cancer Inst., 24, 463

Lam, J. (1956a) Isolation and identification of 3,4-benzpyrene, chrysene, and a number of other aromatic hydrocarbons in the pyrolysis products from dicetyl. Acta path. microbiol. scand., 39, 198

Lam, J. (1956b) Determination of 3,4-benzpyrene and other aromatic compounds formed by pyrolysis of aliphatic tobacco hydrocarbons. Acta path. microbiol. scand., 39, 207

Lijinsky, W. & Raha, C.R. (1961) Polycyclic aromatic hydrocarbons in commercial solvents. Toxicol. appl. Pharmacol., 3, 469

Lijinsky, W. & Ross, A.E. (1967) Production of carcinogenic polynuclear hydrocarbons in the cooking of food. Food cosmet. Toxicol., 5, 343

Lijinsky, W. & Shubik, P. (1965a) Polynuclear hydrocarbon carcinogens in cooked meat and smoked food. Industr. Med. Surg., 34, 152

Lijinsky, W. & Shubik, P. (1965b) The detection of polycyclic aromatic hydrocarbons in liquid smoke and some foods. Toxicol. appl. Pharmacol., 7, 337

Lijinsky, W., Raha, C.R. & Keeling, J. (1961) Comparison of procedures for the determination of polycyclic aromatic hydrocarbons in waxes. Analyt. Chem., 33, 810

Lijinsky, W., Domsky, I., Mason, G., Ramahi, H.Y. & Safavi, T. (1963) The chromatographic determination of trace amounts of polynuclear hydrocarbons in petrolatum, mineral oil, and coal tar. Analyt. Chem., 35, 952

Long, R. & Tompkins, E.E. (1967) Formation of polycyclic aromatic hydrocarbons in pre-mixed acetylene-oxygen flames. Nature (Lond.), 213, 1011

Malanoski, A.J., Greenfield, E.L., Barnes, C.J., Worthington, J.M. & Joe, F.L. (1968) Survey of polycyclic aromatic hydrocarbons in smoked foods. J. Ass. off. analyt. Chem., 51, 114

Masuda, Y. & Kuratsune, M. (1971) Polycyclic aromatic hydrocarbons in smoked fish, "katsuobushi". Gann, 62, 27

Masuda, Y., Mori, K., Hirohata, T. & Kuratsune, M. (1966a) Carcinogenesis in the esophagus. III. Polycyclic aromatic hydrocarbons and phenols in whisky. Gann, 57, 549

Masuda, Y., Mori, K. & Kuratsune, M. (1966b) Polycyclic aromatic hydrocarbons in common Japanese foods. I. Broiled fish, roasted barley, shoyu, and caramel. Gann, 57, 133

Masuda, Y., Mori, K. & Kuratsune, M. (1967) Polycyclic aromatic hydrocarbons formed by pyrolysis of carbohydrates, amino acids and fatty acids. Gann, 58, 69

Ouchi, K. & Imuta, K. (1963) The analysis of benzene extracts of Yubari coal. II. Analysis by gas chromatography. Fuel, 42, 445

Reckner, L.R., Scott, W.E. & Biller, W.F. (1965) The composition and odor of diesel exhaust. Proc. amer. petrol. Inst., 45, 133

Rhee, K.S. & Bratzler, L.J. (1968) Polycyclic hydrocarbon composition of wood smoke. J. food Sci., 33, 626

Riegel, B., Wartman, W.B., Hill, W.T., Reeb, B.B., Shubik, P. & Stanger, D.W. (1951) Delay of methylcholanthrene skin carcinogenesis in mice by 1,2,5,6-dibenzofluorene. Cancer Res., 11, 301

Sawicki, E. (1964) The separation and analysis of polynuclear aromatic hydrocarbons present in the human environment. I-III. Chemist-Analyst, 53, 24, 56, 88

Sawicki, E., Elbert, W., Stanley, T.W., Hauser, T.R. & Fox, F.T. (1960a) Separation and characterization of polynuclear aromatic hydrocarbons in urban air-borne particulates. Analyt. Chem., 32, 810

Sawicki, E., Hauser, T.R. & Stanley, T.W. (1960b) Ultraviolet, visible and fluorescence spectral analysis of polynuclear hydrocarbons. Int. J. air Pollut., 2, 253

Sawicki, E., Meeker, J.E. & Morgan, M.J. (1965) The quantitative composition of air pollution source effluents in terms of aza heterocyclic compounds and polynuclear aromatic hydrocarbons. Int. J. air wat. Pollut., 9, 291

Sawicki, E., Corey, R.C., Dooley, A.E., Gisclard, J.B., Monkmann, J.L., Neligan, R.E. & Ripperton, L.A. (1970) Tentative method of analysis for polynuclear aromatic hydrocarbon content of atmospheric particulate matter. Hlth lab. Sci., 7, Suppl., 31

Schaad, R. (1970) Chromatographie (karzinogener) polyzyklischer aromatischer Kohlenwasserstoffe. Chromat. Rev., 13, 61

Schoental, R. & Scott, E.J.Y. (1949) Fluorescence spectra of polycyclic aromatic hydrocarbons in solution. J. chem. Soc., 1683

Schürch, O. & Winterstein, A. (1935) Über die krebserregende Wirkung aromatischer Kohlenwasserstoffe. Hoppe-Seylers Z. physiol. Chem., 236, 79

Searl, T.D., Cassidy, F.J., King, W.H. & Brown, R.A. (1970) An analytical method for polynuclear aromatic compounds in coke oven effluents by combined use of gas chromatography and ultraviolet absorption spectrometry. Analyt. Chem., 42, 954

Shear, M.J. & Leiter, J. (1941) Studies in carcinogenesis. XVI. Production of subcutaneous tumors in mice by miscellaneous polycyclic compounds. J. nat. Cancer Inst., 2, 241

Sims, P. (1970) Qualitative and quantitative studies on the metabolism of a series of aromatic hydrocarbons by rat-liver preparations. Biochem. Pharmacol., 19, 795

Stefanescu, A. & Stanescu, L. (1968) Der Gefährdungsgrad unter Einwirkung der aromatischen polynuklearen Kohlenwasserstoffe beim Fabrikationsprozess von Russ. II. Die Gefährdung durch einige krebserzeugende Kohlenwasserstoffe und ihre Bestimmung in der Luft. Z. ges. Hyg., 14, 599

Steiner, P.E. (1955) Carcinogenicity of multiple chemicals simultaneously administered. Cancer Res., 15, 632

Steiner, P.E. & Falk, H.L. (1951) Summation and inhibition effects of weak and strong carcinogenic hydrocarbons: 1,2-benzanthracene, chrysene, 1,2,5,6-dibenzanthracene and 20-methylcholanthrene. Cancer Res., 11, 56

Tóth, L. (1971) Polyzyklische Kohlenwasserstoffe in geräuchertem Schinken und Bauchspeck. Fleischwirtschaft, 7, 1069

Tye, R., Burton, M.J., Bingham, E., Bell, Z. & Horton, A.W. (1966a) Carcinogens in a cracked petroleum residuum. Arch. environ. Hlth, 13, 202

Tye, R., Horton, A.W. & Rapien, I. (1966b) Benzo(a)pyrene and other aromatic hydrocarbons extractable from bituminous coal. Amer. industr. Hyg. Ass. J., 27, 25

Van Duuren, B.L. (1958) The polynuclear aromatic hydrocarbons in cigarette-smoke condensate. II. J. nat. Cancer Inst., 21, 623

Van Duuren, B.L., Sivak, A., Segal, A., Orris, L. & Langseth, L. (1966) The tumor-promoting agents of tobacco leaf and tobacco smoke condensate. J. nat. Cancer Inst., 37, 519

Wallcave, L., Garcia, H., Feldman, R., Lijinsky, W. & Shubik, P. (1971) Skin tumorigenesis in mice by petroleum asphalts and coal-tar pitches of known polynuclear aromatic hydrocarbon content. Toxicol. appl. Pharmacol., 18, 41

Wynder, E.L. & Hoffmann, D. (1959) A study of tobacco carcinogenesis. VII. The role of higher polycyclic hydrocarbons. Cancer, 12, 1079

Wynder, E.L. & Hoffmann, D. (1963) Ein experimenteller Beitrag zur Tabakrauchkanzerogenese. Dtsch. med. Wschr., 88, 623

DIBENZ(a,h)ANTHRACENE*

1. Chemical and Physical Data

1.1 Synonyms

Chem. Abstr. No.: 53-70-3

1,2,5,6-Dibenzanthracene; 1,2,7,8-Dibenzanthracene;
Dibenzo(a,h)anthracene; DB(a,h)A

1.2 Molecular weight and chemical formula

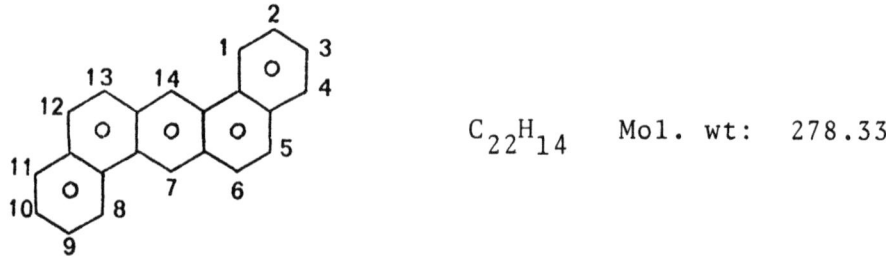

$C_{22}H_{14}$ Mol. wt: 278.33

1.3 Chemical and physical properties of the pure substance

(a) Description: Colourless plates or leaflets from acetic acid. Solution in concentrated sulphuric acid is red. General description in Beilsteins handbook, and in Clar (1964).

(b) Melting-point: 266.5-267°C; 267.5°C; 269-270°C

(c) Density: 1.282

(d) Absorption spectroscopy: The ultra-violet absorption spectrum is described in Perkampus et al. (1967), in heptane; by Clar (1964), in dioxane; and by

---

* Considered by the Working Group in Lyon, December 1972.

Howard et al. (1966b). The infra-red absorption spectrum is described by Pouchert (1970); the nuclear magnetic resonance spectrum by Clin & Lemanceau (1970) and by Haigh & Mallion (1970); and the electron spin resonance spectrum by Brinen (1968).

(e) <u>Identity and purity test</u>: Dibenz(a,h)anthracene (DB(a,h)A) forms a picrate (reddish needles from benzene, melting-point 214°C); a complex with choleic acid (melting-point 221.5-222.3°C, from dioxane); and a complex with 1,3,5-trinitrobenzene (melting-point 237-238.5°C).

(f) <u>Solubility and/or volatility</u>: 0.0005 mg/l dissolve in water at 27°C (Davis et al., 1942). It is soluble in most organic solvents and oils and slightly soluble in alcohol and ether. The distribution coefficient in the nitromethane/cyclohexane system was determined as 1.99 by Müller et al. (1967) and as 2 by Grimmer (1961). DB(a,h)A is sublimable.

(g) <u>Chemical reactivity</u>: In benzene/ether DB(a,h)A adds two atoms of Li or Na with the formation of blue compounds which yield methanol, 7,14-dihydro-dibenz-(a,h)anthracene (Bachmann, 1936) and with CO_2 the corresponding dicarboxylic acid (Bachmann & Pence, 1937). Reduction with Na gives the octa-hydro derivative. DB(a,h)A can be oxidized by chromic acid to dibenz(a,h)anthra-7,14-quinone (Clar, 1929) and further to anthraquinone-1,2,5,6-tetracarboxylic acid (Cook, 1931), and by osmium tetroxide to 5,6-dihydro-5,6-dihydroxy-dibenz(a,h)anthracene and further to dibenz(a,h)anthra-5,6-quinone (Cook & Schoental, 1948; Stephenson, 1949). Electrophilic substitutions occur mainly in position 9.

2. Use and Occurrence

(a) Analytical methods

Several chromatographic procedures for the separation of DB(a,h)A from other substances and for its spectroscopic determination have been published and are extensively reviewed by Sawicki (1964) and by Schaad (1970). They include paper chromatography; column chromatography; thin-layer chromatography (Keefer, 1967; Chatot et al., 1969; Hood & Winefordner, 1968), used for detection in oil (Howard et al., 1966a); gas chromatography (Bhatia, 1971; Chatot et al., 1969; Fryčka, 1972), used for detection in cigarette smoke (Davis, 1969); gel chromatography (Edstrom & Petro, 1968), used for detection in cigarette smoke (Stedman et al., 1968); and ultra-violet absorption spectroscopy or low-temperature fluorescence (Hood & Winefordner, 1968). References to analytical methods used for detection in various media such as air, soil, food, etc., can be found in the section on "Occurrence".

(b) Occurrence

Exhaust: 2.5 mg/kg of exhaust tar were isolated from first run gasoline engine exhaust, and 0.16 from automobile exhaust gas after a one-minute run (Hoffmann & Wynder, 1962a,b, 1963).

Air: According to two review articles (Kotin & Falk, 1963; Sawicki, 1967) DB(a,h)A was not detected among the polycyclic aromatic hydrocarbons found in polluted air. However, the dust of 12 German cities during the month of February contained 3.2-32 µg/1000 m^3 (Grimmer, 1968), and tunnel dust 4-39 µg/kg (Grimmer & Hildebrandt, 1965a).

Cigarette smoke: In the smoke condensate of 100 cigarettes 0.05 (Van Duuren, 1958) - 0.4 µg (Wynder & Hoffmann, 1963) were found, and 0.1-0.15 mg/kg (Elmenhorst & Grimmer, 1968; Wynder & Hoffmann, 1959) were detected in cigarette smoke condensate.

Pyrolysis: DB(a,h)A is formed on pyrolysis of the tobacco constituent stigmasterol (400 mg/kg) at 700°C (Badger et al., 1965).

Occupational exposure: In soot, concentrations ranging from 64-705 mg/1000 m^3 have been detected (Stefanescu & Stanescu, 1968), and coal-tar contained between 230-300 mg/kg (Lijinsky et al., 1963).

Soil: In soil samples in Iceland (lava and humus), concentrations ranged from 0-2.3 µg/kg; and 351 µg/kg have been found in an airfield sample (Grimmer et al., 1972).

Food: DB(a,h)A has been detected in smoked ham (Hamm & Tóth, 1970), and 0.2 µg/kg were found in charcoal-broiled steak (Lijinsky & Shubik, 1964, 1965). In vegetables, the following amounts of DB(a,h)A were found: salad, 0.6-1 µg/kg; kale, 0.1-2.6 µg/kg; spinach, 0.3 µg/kg; tomatoes, 0.04 µg/kg (Grimmer & Hildebrandt, 1965c; Hettche, 1971). In different kinds of refined vegetable oils, concentrations ranged from 0-3 µg/kg (Biernoth & Rost, 1967, 1968), and in crude vegetable oils from 0-1.9 µg/kg, the highest value being found in coconut oil (Grimmer & Hildebrandt, 1967). In coconut fat from smoke-dried copra, between 0.9-4 µg/kg have been found (Biernoth & Rost, 1968). Cereals contained between 0.1-0.6 µg/kg, depending on their source (Grimmer & Hildebrandt, 1965b). In only one out of nine samples of yeast could 0.9 µg/kg be detected (Grimmer & Wilhelm, 1969).

3. Biological Data Relevant to the Evaluation of Carcinogenic Risk to Man

3.1 Carcinogenicity and related studies in animals

DB(a,h)A was the first pure chemical compound shown to be carcinogenic (Kennaway, 1930).

(_a_) Oral administration

Mouse: The addition of DB(a,h)A to food for a total dose of 9-19 mg over a period of five to seven months led to the appearance of tumours of the forestomach in seven out of 22 survivors after one year; one of these tumours was a carcinoma (Larionow & Soboleva, 1938). In a later experiment, 20 A backcross mice receiving 0.4 mg DB(a,h)A/day in a mineral oil emulsion which replaced the drinking-water developed two squamous cell carcinomas and 11 papillomas of the forestomach within 406 days (Lorenz & Stewart, 1948). In similar experiments in which NaOH was used as the emulsifying agent, tumours were produced in the lung, heart and intestine. Squamous carcinomas of the forestomach were induced if the emulsion was stabilized against the breaking effect of gastric juices (Lorenz & Stewart, 1947; Snell & Stewart, 1962). In a study on 42 DBA/2 mice receiving 0.2 mg/ml of olive oil emulsion in the place of drinking-water at an average dose of 0.76-0.85 mg/day, 27/27 survivors at 200 days had pulmonary adenomatosis, 24 had alveologenic carcinoma of the lung, and 16 had haemangio-endotheliomas. In addition 12/13 females had mammary carcinomas. In 35 controls, no mammary tumours and two pulmonary adenomatoses were seen (Snell & Stewart, 1962).

A single dose of 1.5 mg DB(a,h)A in polyethylene glycol-400 produced papillomas of the forestomach in two out of 42 Swiss male mice within 30 weeks (Berenblum & Haran, 1955).

In a series of studies on DB(a,h)A given by stomach tube to mice of several strains, twice weekly administrations of 0.5% DB(a,h)A in almond oil for 15 weeks (total dose, 15 mg) produced mammary carcinomas in one out of 20 intact BALB/c female mice and in 13/24 pseudo-pregnant female BALB/c mice (Biancifiori & Caschera, 1962).

(b) Skin application

Mouse: Many studies on the induction of skin tumours with DB(a,h)A have been reported since that of Kennaway (1930). In C3H (Jax) mice painted twice weekly with 0.25% DB(a,h)A in thiophene-free benzene for life span, 10/11 developed mammary tumours, whereas the incidence in controls which had not been painted was 50% (Ranadive & Karande, 1963). Bi-weekly painting with a 0.2% solution of DB(a,h)A in acetone-benzene (38 µg/dose) of 20 Swiss mice induced skin tumours in 16 animals (Lijinsky et al., 1965).

A dose-response study with thrice weekly paintings of different concentrations of DB(a,h)A in acetone is available on ICR/Ha Swiss mice. Mice which developed tumours following painting with 0.001%, 0.01% and 0.1% solutions were, respectively, one out of 30 (one carcinoma), 43/50 (39 carcinomas), and 39/40 (32 carcinomas). The latent period was also dose related (Van Duuren et al., 1967).

DB(a,h)A can also initiate skin carcinogenesis in mice at doses of as little as 0.02 µg given once (Klein, 1960).

In another experiment on Swiss mice run parallel to a study with benzo(a)pyrene (B(a)P), the carcinogenic strength of the two chemicals was shown to be similar: repeated paintings with a 0.001% solution of B(a)P in acetone produced papillomas in 43% and carcinomas in 3% of the mice, and the same concentration of DB(a,h)A produced papillomas in 30% and carcinomas in 30%. On the other hand, a 0.01% solution of either compound produced both papillomas and carcinomas in over 90% of mice, with similar latent periods (Wynder & Hoffmann, 1959).

Hamster: No tumours were seen among 10 Syrian golden hamsters receiving 20 applications of a 0.2% solution of DB(a,h)A in mineral oil over a period of 10 weeks, five of which were alive at 50 weeks (Shubik et al., 1960).

(c) Inhalation and/or intratracheal administration

Rat: A total of 170 rats received five intratracheal administrations of a suspension of DB(a,h)A in protein blood substitute BK-8 with finely powdered black India ink for a total dose of either 0, 0.5, 2, 10 or 20 mg DB(a,h)A and were observed for 30 months. Ratios of animals with lung squamous cell carcinomas/survivors at the appearance of first tumour or at the end of experiment were, respectively, 0/15, 0/18, 1/27, 4/21 and 6/13 (Yanysheva & Balenko, 1966).

(d) Subcutaneous and/or intramuscular administration

Mouse: Many experiments have been performed (Hartwell, 1951; Shubik & Hartwell, 1957, 1969; Thompson & Co., 1971). The most significant dose-response study is still that of Bryan & Shimkin (1943) in which DB(a,h)A dissolved in tricaprylin was given to groups of at least 19 C3H mice as a single injection. At doses of 0.00019, 0.0078, 0.016, 0.03, 0.06, 0.12, 0.25, 0.5, 1, 2, 4 or 8 mg the respective incidence of local sarcomas was 2/79, 6/40, 6/19, 16/21, 20/20, 21/23, 19/21, 20/21, 22/22, 19/19, 17/20 and 16/21. Thus, the lowest effective dose of DB(a,h)A was 0.0019 mg, whereas 3-methylcholanthrene (MC) did not induce tumours at doses of 0.0039 mg or lower. Considering together all mice receiving 0.0019-0.031 mg, DB(a,h)A induced sarcomas in 30/159, whereas B(a)P did so in two out of 156. However, average minimal latent periods were 3.7 months for DB(a,h)A, two to five months for MC and three for B(a)P.

The same order of magnitude for the effective doses of DB(a,h)A had been observed in a previous study in an unspecified strain of mice (Dobrovolskaia-Zavadskaia, 1938). In another study, a total of 0.0125 mg DB(a,h)A in lard given as five injections induced sarcomas in four of 20 mice (Lettinga, 1937). The number of lung adenomas was increased in some studies following s.c. injection.

Newborn mouse: A dose-response relationship has been established among groups of General Purpose/NIH newborn mice receiving subcutaneous injections of logarithmically spaced dose levels ranging between 0.003 and 6.7 µg/mouse. At 0.08 µg and above, a consistent, dose related appearance of local sarcomas was observed. The incidence of lung adenomas increased at 0.2 µg and above. This study was run in parallel to experiments with MC, and it appears that DB(a,h)A was more active than MC. Sarcomas at the injection site were seen sporadically following administration of

0.003-0.01 µg DB(a,h)A, and consistently at 0.08 µg and above, whereas MC induced sarcomas only at 0.4 µg and above. Similarly, an increase in lung adenomas was detected for 0.2 µg DB(a,h)A and for 1.2 µg MC (O'Gara et al., 1965).

Rat: When DB(a,h)A dissolved in lard was given as four injections of 8 mg at monthly intervals, 11 of an original number of 40 rats developed tumours in the course of a year (Shear, 1936). Single doses of 0.1 mg or 1 mg in olive oil produced sarcomas, respectively, in three out of nine and in six out of 10 rats (Roussy et al., 1942).

Guinea pig: Multiple s.c. injections of total doses of 8-48 mg DB(a,h)A in sunflower seed oil produced two sarcomas (the first at 19 months) out of an original number of 25 animals (Shabad, 1938; Shabad & Urinson, 1938).

Pigeon: Of 121 pigeons which received intramuscular injections of 3 mg DB(a,h)A in benzene and were observed for 13 months, 14 developed a fibrosarcoma at the injection site. No tumours were found among 32 untreated controls (Prichard et al., 1964).

Fowl: Intramuscular injection of 0.4% DB(a,h)A in lard induced sarcomas in 15/31 fowl within 45 months (Peacock, 1935).

(e) Other experimental systems

Pulmonary administration: Lung adenomas in mice have occurred following different routes of administration and also following direct administration into the lung through the chest wall (Andervont, 1937;

Rask-Nielson, 1950; Kuschner et al., 1956). A dose-response relationship has been found following single intravenous injections of DB(a,h)A to A mice as a colloidal dispersion in water. The percentage of lung-tumour bearing animals and the number of lung adenomas per mouse increased with increasing dose. The lowest dose used was 0.1 mg/mouse, and this increased both the parameters considered (Heston & Schneidermann, 1953).

<u>Intrarenal injection</u>: The injection of 0.3-0.5 mg DB(a,h)A in olive oil into the kidney of <u>frogs</u> (<u>Rana pipiens</u>) produced renal adenocarcinomas in 26% of the survivors compared with 3% of the controls (Strauss & Mateyko, 1964).

3.2 Other relevant biological data

Some hydroxylated metabolites of DB(a,h)A have been detected in experimental systems (Boyland & Sims, 1965; Sims, 1970). K-region epoxide and <u>cis</u>-dihydrodiol derivatives from DB(a,h)A have been found to be more active in the production of malignant transformation in hamster embryo cells than the hydrocarbon or the corresponding K-region phenol (Grover et al., 1971).

3.3 Observations in man

None were available to the Working Group.

4. Comments on Data Reported and Evaluation

4.1 Animal data

DB(a,h)A has produced tumours by different routes of administration in mice, rats, guinea pigs, frogs, pigeons and chickens. It has both local and systemic carcinogenic effects.

On oral administration, it produced tumours of the forestomach in the mouse; intratracheal administration to hamsters produced lung tumours.

In repeated skin painting experiments in mice, DB(a,h)A and B(a)P appeared to be equally effective. In a dose-response study on s.c. carcinogenicity with DB(a,h)A, B(a)P and MC, DB(a,h)A was shown to be effective at a lower dose than that effective for B(a)P or for MC; its latent period, however, was longer. DB(a,h)A induced local sarcomas and increased the incidence of lung adenomas following a single s.c. injection in newborn mice at dose levels which were ineffective with MC.

It has not been adequately tested in other species.

4.2 Human data

No case reports or epidemiological studies on the significance of DB(a,h)A exposure to man are available. However, coal-tar and other materials which are known to be carcinogenic to man may contain DB(a,h)A. The substance has also been detected in other environmental situations. The possible contribution of polycyclic aromatic hydrocarbons from some environmental sources to the overall carcinogenic risk to man is discussed in the preamble.

5. References

Andervont, H.B. (1937) Pulmonary tumours in mice. I. The susceptibility of the lungs of albino mice to the carcinogenic action of 1,2,5,6-dibenzanthracene. Publ. Hlth Rep. (Wash.), 52, 212

Bachmann, W.E. (1936) The reaction of alkalimetals with polycyclic hydrocarbons: 1,2-benzanthracene, 1,2,5,6-dibenzanthracene and methylcholanthrene. J. org. Chem., 1, 347

Bachmann, W.E. & Pence, L.H. (1937) The reaction of alkali metals with polycyclic hydrocarbons. J. amer. chem. Soc., 59, 2339

Badger, G.M., Donnelly, J.K. & Spotswood, T.M. (1965) The formation of aromatic hydrocarbons at high temperatures. XXIV. The pyrolysis of some tobacco constitutents. Aust. J. Chem., 18, 1249

Beilsteins Handbuch der Organischen Chemie, 5, III, 2553

Berenblum, I. & Haran, N. (1955) The influence of croton oil and of polyethylene glycol-400 on carcinogenesis in the forestomach of the mouse. Cancer Res., 15, 510

Bhatia, K. (1971) Gas chromatographic determination of polycyclic aromatic hydrocarbons. Analyt. Chem., 43, 609

Biancifiori, C. & Caschera, F. (1962) The relation between pseudopregnancy and the chemical induction by four carcinogens of mammary and ovarian tumours in BALB/c mice. Brit. J. Cancer, 16, 722

Biernoth, G. & Rost, H.E. (1967) The occurrence of polycyclic aromatic hydrocarbons in coconut oil and their removal. Chem. and Ind., 2002

Biernoth, G. & Rost, H.E. (1968) Vorkommen polycyclischer aromatischer Kohlenwasserstoffe in Speiseölen und deren Entfernung. Arch. Hyg. (Muenchen), 152, 238

Boyland, E. & Sims, P. (1965) The metabolism of benz(a)anthracene and dibenz(a,h)anthracene and their 5,6-epoxy-5,6-dihydro derivatives by rat liver homogenates. Biochem. J., 97, 7

Brinen, J.S. (1968) ESR studies of organic triplet states. Extinction coefficients of T-T' transitions. In: Lim, E.C., ed., International Conference on Molecular Luminescence, Chicago, New York, Amsterdam, W.A. Benjamin, p. 333

Bryan, W.R. & Shimkin, M.B. (1943) Quantitative analysis of dose-response data obtained with three carcinogenic hydrocarbons in strain C_3H male mice. J. nat. Cancer Inst., 3, 503

Chatot, G., Jequier, W., Jay, M., Fontages, R. & Obaton, P. (1969) Atmospheric polycyclic hydrocarbons. I. Problems connected with the coupling of thin-layer chromatography and gas chromatography. J. Chromat., 45, 415

Clar, E. (1929) Zur Kenntnis mehrkerniger aromatischer Kohlenwasserstoffe und ihrer Abkömmlinge. I. Dibenzanthracene und ihre Chinone. Ber. dtsch. chem. Ges., 62, 350

Clar, E. (1964) Polycyclic hydrocarbons, Vol. 1, London, New York, Academic Press; Berlin, Göttingen, Heidelberg, Springer-Verlag, p. 337

Clin, B. & Lemanceau, B. (1970) Nuclear magnetic resonance study of carcinogenic and noncarcinogenic isomers (dibenzacridines and dibenzanthracenes). C.R. Acad. Sci. (Paris), Ser. D, 271, 788

Cook, J.W. (1931) Polycyclic aromatic hydrocarbons. VIII. The chemistry of 1,2,5,6-dibenzanthracene. J. chem. Soc., 3273

Cook, J.W. & Schoental, R. (1948) Oxidation of carcinogenic hydrocarbons by osmium tetroxide. J. chem. Soc., 170

Davis, H.J. (1969) Gas-chromatographic display of the polycyclic aromatic hydrocarbon fraction of cigarette smoke. Talanta, 16, 621

Davis, W.W., Krahl, M.E. & Clowes, G.H.A. (1942) Solubility of carcinogenic and related hydrocarbons in water. J. amer. chem. Soc., 64, 108

Dobrovolskaia-Zavadskaia, N. (1938) Les doses minimes de 1,2,5,6-dibenzanthracène capables de produire, en une seule injection sous-cutanée, un cancer chez la souris. C.R. Soc. Biol. (Paris), 129, 1055

Edstrom, T. & Petro, B.A. (1968) Gel permeation chromatographic studies of polynuclear aromatic hydrocarbon materials. J. polymer Sci. C, 21, 171

Elmenhorst, H. & Grimmer, G. (1968) Polycyclische Kohlenwasserstoffe aus Zigarettenrauchenkondensat. Eine Methode zur Fraktionierung grosser Mengen für Tierversuche. Z. Krebsforsch., 71, 66

Fryčka, J. (1972) Separation of polynuclear aromatic hydrocarbons by gas-solid chromatography on graphitized carbon black deposited on chromosorb W. J. Chromat., 65, 432

Grimmer, G. (1961) Eine Methode zur Bestimmung von 3,4-Benzpyren in Tabakrauchkondensaten. Beitr. Tabakforsch., 1, 107

Grimmer, G. (1968) Cancerogene Kohlenwasserstoffe in der Umgebung des Menschen. Dtsch. Apoth. Ztg, 108, 529

Grimmer, G. & Hildebrandt, A. (1965a) Kohlenwasserstoffe in der Umgebung des Menschen. I. Eine Methode zur simultanen Bestimmung von dreizehn polycyclischen Kohlenwasserstoffen. J. Chromat., 20, 89

Grimmer, G. & Hildebrandt, A. (1965b) Kohlenwasserstoffe in der Umgebung des Menschen. II. Der Gehalt polycyclischer Kohlenwasserstoffe in Brotgetreide verschiedener Standorte. Z. Krebsforsch., 67, 272

Grimmer, G. & Hildebrandt, A. (1965c) Kohlenwasserstoffe in der Umgebung des Menschen. III. Der Gehalt polycyclischer Kohlenwasserstoffe in verschiedenen Gemüsesorten und Salaten. Dtsch. Lebensmitt.-Rdsch., 61, 272

Grimmer, G. & Hildebrandt, A. (1967) Content of polycyclic hydrocarbons in crude vegetable oils. Chem. and Ind., 2000

Grimmer, G. & Wilhelm, G. (1969) Der Gehalt von polycyclischen Kohlenwasserstoffe in europäischen Hefen. Dtsch. Lebensmitt.-Rdsch., 65, 229

Grimmer, G., Jacob, J. & Hildebrandt, A. (1972) Kohlenwasserstoffe in der Umgebung des Menschen. IX. Der Gehalt polycyclischer Kohlenwasserstoffe in isländischen Bodenproben. Z. Krebsforsch., 78, 65

Grover, P.L., Sims, P., Huberman, E., Marquardt, H., Kuroki, T. & Heidelberger, C. (1971) In vitro transformation of rodent cells by K-region derivatives of polycyclic hydrocarbons. Proc. nat. Acad. Sci. (Wash.), 689, 1098

Haigh, C.W. & Mallion, R.B. (1970) Proton magnetic resonance of planar condensed benzenoid hydrocarbons. I. Analysis of spectra. Molec. Phys., 18, 737

Hamm, R. & Tóth, L. (1970) Cancerogene Kohlenwasserstoffe in geräucherten Fleischerzeugnissen. *Med. u. Ehnähr.*, 11, 25

Hartwell, J.L. (1951) *Survey of compounds which have been tested for carcinogenic activity*, Washington, D.C., Government Printing Office (Public Health Service Publication No. 149)

Heston, W.E. & Schneidermann, M.A. (1953) Analysis of dose-response in relation to mechanism of pulmonary tumor induction in mice. *Science*, 117, 109

Hettche, H.O. (1971) Plant waxes as collectors of polycyclic aromatics in the air of residential areas. *Staub (Engl. Transl.)*, 31, 34

Hoffmann, D. & Wynder, E.L. (1962a) A study of air pollution carcinogenesis. II. The isolation and identification of polynuclear aromatic hydrocarbons from gasoline engine exhaust condensate. *Cancer*, 15, 93

Hoffmann, D. & Wynder, E.L. (1962b) Analytical and biological studies on gasoline engine exhaust. *Nat. Cancer Inst. Monogr.*, 9, 91

Hoffmann, D. & Wynder, E.L. (1963) Studies on gasoline engine exhaust. *J. air Pollut. Control Ass.*, 13, 322

Hood, L.V.S. & Winefordner, J.D. (1968) Thin-layer separation and low-temperature luminescence measurement of mixtures of carcinogens. *Analyt. Chim. Acta*, 42, 199

Howard, J.W., Teague, R.T., White, R.H. & Fry, B.E. (1966a) Extraction and estimation of polycyclic aromatic hydrocarbons in smoked foods. I. General method. *J. Ass. off. analyt. Chem.*, 49, 595

Howard, J.W., Turicchi, E.W., White, R.H. & Fazio, T. (1966b) Extraction and estimation of polycyclic aromatic hydrocarbons in vegetable oil. *J. Ass. off. analyt. Chem.*, 49, 1236

Keefer, L.K. (1967) Magnesium hydroxide as a thin-layer chromatographic adsorbent. A new system for the separation of polynuclear hydrocarbons. *J. Chromat.*, 31, 390

Kennaway, E.L. (1930) Further experiments on cancer producing substances. Biochem. J., 24, 497

Klein, M. (1960) A comparison of the initiating and promoting actions of 9,10-dimethyl-1,2-benzanthracene and 1,2,5,6-dibenzanthracene in skin tumorigenesis. Cancer Res., 20, 1179

Kotin, P. & Falk, H. (1963) Atmospheric factors in pathogenesis of lung cancer. Advanc. Cancer Res., 7, 475

Kuschner, M., Laskin, S., Cristofano, E. & Nelson, N. (1956) Experimental carcinoma of the lung. In: Proceedings of the Third National Cancer Conference, Detroit, Philadelphia, Montreal, Lippincott, p. 485

Larionow, L.F. & Soboleva, N.G. (1938) Gastric tumors experimentally produced in mice by means of benzopyrene and dibenzanthracene. Vestn. Rentgenol. Radiol., 20, 276

Lettinga, T.W. (1937) De carcinogene werking van kleine doses 1,2,5,6-dibenzanthraceen. (MD Thesis, Amsterdam)

Lijinsky, W. & Ross, A.E. (1967) Production of carcinogenic polynuclear hydrocarbons in the cooking of food. Food cosmet. Toxicol., 5, 343

Lijinsky, W. & Shubik, P. (1964) Benzo(a)pyrene and other polynuclear hydrocarbons in charcoal-broiled meat. Science, 145, 53

Lijinsky, W. & Shubik, P. (1965) Polynuclear hydrocarbon carcinogens in cooked meat and smoked food. Industr. Med. Surg., 34, 152

Lijinsky, W., Domsky, I., Mason, G., Ramahi, H.Y. & Safavi, T. (1963) The chromatographic determination of trace amounts of polynuclear hydrocarbons in petrolatum, mineral oil and coal-tar. Analyt. Chem., 35, 952

Lijinsky, W., Garcia, H., Terracini, B. & Saffiotti, U. (1965) Tumorigenic activity of hydrogenated derivatives of dibenz(a,h)anthracene. J. nat. Cancer Inst., 34, 1

Lorenz, E. & Stewart, H.L. (1947) Tumours of alimentary tract induced in mice by feeding olive oil emulsions containing carcinogenic hydrocarbons. J. nat. Cancer Inst., 7, 227

Lorenz, E. & Stewart, H.L. (1948) Tumours of alimentary tract in mice fed carcinogenic hydrocarbons in mineral oil emulsions. J. nat. Cancer Inst., 9, 173

Müller, R., Moldenhauer, W. & Schlemmer, P. (1967) Erfahrungen bei der quantitativen Bestimmung von polycyclischen Kohlenwasserstoffen im Tabakrauch. Ber. Inst. Tabakforsch. (Dresden), 14, 159

O'Gara, R.W., Kelly, M.G., Brown, J. & Mantel, N. (1965) Induction of tumors in mice given a minute single dose of dibenz-(a,h)anthracene or 3-methylcholanthrene as newborns. A dose-response study. J. nat. Cancer Inst., 35, 1027

Peacock, P.R. (1935) Studies of fowl tumours induced by carcinogenic agents. Amer. J. Cancer, 25, 37

Perkampus, H.H., Sandeman, I. & Timmons, C.J., eds. (1967) DMS UV Atlas of Organic Compounds, Vol. III, Weinheim, Verlag Chemie; London, Butterworths, E5/6

Pouchert, C.J., ed. (1970) Aldrich Library of Infrared Spectra, Milwaukee, Wisc., Aldrich Chemical Co. Inc., p. 439

Prichard, R.W., Eubanks, J.W. & Hazlett, C.C. (1964) Age and breed effects on induction of sarcomas by dibenz(a,h)-anthracene in pigeons. J. nat. Cancer Inst., 32, 905

Ranadive, K.J. & Karande, K.A. (1963) Studies on 1,2,5,6-dibenzanthracene-induced mammary carcinogenesis in mice. Brit. J. Cancer, 17, 272

Rask-Nielsen, R. (1950) The susceptibility of the thymus, lung, subcutaneous and mammary tissues in strain street mice to direct application of small doses of four different carcinogenic hydrocarbons. Brit. J. Cancer, 4, 108

Roussy, G., Guérin, M. & Guérin, P. (1942) Activité comparée des trois principaux hydrocarbures synthétiques cancérigènes. Bull. Cancer, 30, 66

Sawicki, E. (1964) The separation and analysis of polynuclear aromatic hydrocarbons present in the human environment. I-III. Chemist-Analyst, 53, 24, 56, 88

Sawicki, E. (1967) Airborne carcinogens and allied compounds. Arch. environ. Hlth, 14, 46

Schaad, R.E. (1970) Chromatographie (karzinogener) polycyclischer aromatischer Kohlenwasserstoffe. Chromat. Rev., 13, 61

Shabad, L.M. (1938) Experimental tumours in guinea pigs. Arh. Biol. Nauk, 51, 112

Shabad, L.M. & Urinson, J.P. (1938) Alterations in the liver of guinea pigs following administration of a chemically pure carcinogenic substance, 1,2,5,6-dibenzanthracene. Arh. Biol. Nauk, 51, 105

Shear, M.J. (1936) Studies in carcinogenesis. I. The production of tumours in mice with hydrocarbons. Amer. J. Cancer, 26, 322

Shubik, P. & Hartwell, J.L. (1957) Survey of compounds which have been tested for carcinogenic activity, Washington, D.C., Government Printing Office (Public Health Service Publication No. 149: Supplement 1)

Shubik, P. & Hartwell, J.L. (1969) Survey of compounds which have been tested for carcinogenic activity, Washington, D.C., Government Printing Office (Public Health Service Publication No. 149: Supplement 2)

Shubik, P., Pietra, G. & Della Porta, G. (1960) Studies of skin carcinogenesis in the Syrian golden hamster. Cancer Res., 20, 100

Sims, P. (1970) Qualitative and quantitative studies on the metabolism of a series of aromatic hydrocarbons by rat-liver preparations. Biochem. Pharmacol., 19, 795

Snell, K.C. & Stewart, H.L. (1962) Pulmonary adenomatosis induced in DBA/2 mice by oral administration of dibenz(a,h)anthracene. J. nat. Cancer Inst., 28, 1043

Stedman, R.L., Miller, R.L., Lakritz, L. & Chamberlain, W.J. (1968) Methods for concentrating polynuclear aromatic hydrocarbons in cigarette smoke condensate. Chem. and Ind., 394

Stefanescu, A. & Stanescu, L. (1968) Der Gefährdungsgrad unter Einwirkung der aromatischen polynuklearen Kohlenwasserstoffe beim Fabrikationsprozess von Russ. II. Die Gefährdung durch einige krebserzeugende Kohlenwasserstoffe und ihre Bestimmung in der Luft. Z. ges. Hyg., 14, 599

Stephenson, E.F.M. (1949) The Schmidt reaction on 1,2,5,6-dibenzanthra-3,4-quinone. *J. chem. Soc.*, 2620

Strauss, E. & Mateyko, G.M. (1964) Chemical induction of neoplasms in the kidney of *Rana pipiens*. *Cancer Res.*, *24*, 1969

Thompson, J.I. & Co. (1971) *Survey of compounds which have been tested for carcinogenic activity*, Washington, D.C., Government Printing Office (Public Health Service Publication No. 149: 1968-1969)

Van Duuren, B.L. (1958) The polynuclear aromatic hydrocarbons in cigarette-smoke condensate. II. *J. nat. Cancer Inst.*, *21*, 623

Van Duuren, B.L., Langseth, L., Goldschmidt, B.M. & Orris, L. (1967) Carcinogenicity of epoxides, lactones and peroxy compounds. VI. Structure and carcinogenic activity. *J. nat. Cancer Inst.*, *39*, 1217

Wynder, E.L. & Hoffmann, D. (1959) A study of tobacco carcinogenesis. VII. The role of higher polycyclic hydrocarbons. *Cancer*, *12*, 1079

Wynder, E.L. & Hoffmann, D. (1963) Ein experimenteller Beitrag zur Tabakrauchkanzerogenese. *Dtsch. med. Wschr.*, *88*, 623

Yanysheva, N.Y. & Balenko, N.V. (1966) Experimental lung cancer caused by introduction of various doses of 1,2,5,6-dibenzanthracene. *Gig. i Sanit.*, *31*, 12

DIBENZO(h,rst)PENTAPHENE*

1. Chemical and Physical Data

1.1 Synonyms

Chem. Abstr. No.: 194-47-2

Tribenzo(a,e,i)pyrene; (1,2,4,5,7,8)-Tribenzopyrene; (1,2,4,5,8,9)-Tribenzopyrene

1.2 Chemical formula and molecular weight

$C_{28}H_{16}$ Mol. wt: 352.44

1.3 Chemical and physical properties of the pure substance

(a) Description: Pale yellow needles from xylene. General description in Beilsteins handbook, and in Clar (1964).

(b) Melting-point: 320-321°C

(c) Absorption spectroscopy: The ultra-violet absorption spectrum, in cyclohexane, is described by Clar (1964) and in cyclohexane or benzene in Perkampus et al. (1967). The maximum of fluorescence

---

* Considered by the Working Group in Lyon, December 1972.

and the relative molar extinction are given by Sawicki et al. (1960) and Sawicki (1969).

(d) <u>Solubility and/or volatility</u>: The substance is soluble in concentrated H_2SO_4. The solution has a green colour which on heating turns red. Solutions in xylene have a blue fluorescence.

(e) <u>Chemical reactivity</u>: Data on π-electron distribution are given by Mallion (1971), and Snyder (1963) reported on the energy of adsorption on Al_2O_3/H_2O.

2. Use and Occurrence

(a) <u>Analytical methods</u>

For the detection of dibenzo(h,rst)pentaphene in air pollutants Matsushita et al. (1970) used as a clean-up step the sublimation at 300°C and 0.01 Torr. Further cleaning and identification is done by thin-layer chromatography and fluorescence spectroscopy.

(b) <u>Occurrence</u>

The compound has been identified in suspended particulate matter from Kawasaki air (Matsushita et al., 1970).

3. Biological Data Relevant to the Evaluation of Carcinogenic Risk to Man

3.1 <u>Carcinogenicity and related studies in animals</u>

(a) <u>Subcutaneous and/or intramuscular administration</u>

<u>Mouse</u>: Twenty-seven XVII/nc/Z mice (eight male, 19 female) were each injected subcutaneously with three

doses of 0.6 mg dibenzo(h,rst)pentaphene in olive oil; three males developed sarcomas after 242-320 days, and six females developed sarcomas after 180-242 days (Lacassagne et al., 1964).

3.2 Other relevant biological data

None were available to the Working Group.

3.3 Observations in man

None were available to the Working Group.

4. Comments on Data Reported and Evaluation

4.1 Animal data

In the only experiment reported, subcutaneous injection in mice induced sarcomas. It has not been tested by other routes in the mouse or in other species.

4.2 Human data

No case reports or epidemiological studies on the significance of dibenzo(h,rst)pentaphene exposure to man are available. Only one study reports its occurrence in urban air.

5. References

Beilsteins Handbuch der Organischen Chemie, 5, III, 2700

Clar, E. (1964) Polycyclic Hydrocarbons, Vol. 2, London, New York, Academic Press; Berlin, Göttingen, Heidelberg, Springer-Verlag, pp. 157, 159

Lacassagne, A., Buu-Hoi, N.P., Zajdela, F. & Lavit-Lamy, D. (1964) Activité cancérogène de dérivés substitués du 1,2,3,4-dibenzopyrène, du 1,2,4,5-dibenzopyrène, et du 1,2,4,5,8,9-tribenzopyrène. C.R. Acad. Sci. (Paris), 259, 3899

Mallion, R.B. (1971) Calculation of the π-electron ring current properties of some carcinogenic, heptacyclic, condensed, benzenoid hydrocarbons. J. med. Chem., 14, 824

Matsushita, H., Esumi, Y. & Yamada, K. (1970) Identification of polynuclear hydrocarbons in air pollutants. Bunseki Kagaku, 19, 951

Perkampus, H.H., Sandeman, I. & Timmons, C.J., eds. (1967) DMS UV Atlas of Organic Compounds, Vol. III, Weinheim, Verlag Chemie; London, Butterworths, E6/17

Sawicki, E. (1969) Fluorescence analysis in air pollution research. Talanta, 16, 1231

Sawicki, E., Hauser, T.R. & Stanley, T.W. (1960) Ultraviolet, visible and fluorescence spectral analysis of polynuclear hydrocarbons. Int. J. air Pollut., 2, 253

Snyder, L.R. (1963) Adsorption from solution. I. Fused aromatic hydrocarbons on aluminia. J. phys. Chem., 67, 234

DIBENZO(a,e)PYRENE*

1. Chemical and Physical Data

1.1 Synonyms

Chem. Abstr. No.: 192-65-4

Chem. Abstr. Name: Naphtho(1,2,3,4,def)chrysene

1,2,4,5-Dibenzopyrene; DB(a,e)P

1.2 Chemical formula and molecular weight

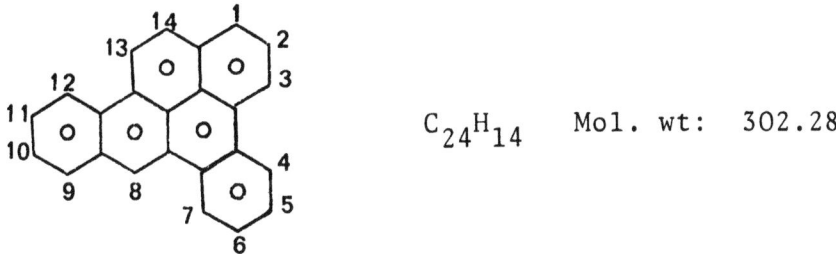

$C_{24}H_{14}$ Mol. wt: 302.28

1.3 Chemical and physical properties of the pure substance

(a) *Description*: Yellow needles from toluene, xylene or chlorobenzene. General description in Beilsteins handbook, and in Clar (1964).

(b) *Melting-point*: 241-242°C, 233-234°C

(c) *Absorption spectroscopy*: The ultraviolet absorption spectrum is described by Clar (1964), in benzene, and by Sawicki et al. (1960); in petrol ether. Lyons (1959) presented data on the fluorescence spectrum, in benzene. The maximum

---

* Considered by the Working Group in Lyon, December 1972.

of fluorescence and the relative molar extinction are given by Sawicki (1969).

(<u>d</u>) <u>Solubility and/or volatility</u>: Solutions in organic solvents are yellow and have a green or blue fluorescence. Concentrated H_2SO_4 solutions have a red colour and a brown fluorescence. Demish & Wright (1963) determined the distribution coefficient between hexane and aqueous monoethanolammoniumdeoxycholate as 6.8.

(<u>e</u>) <u>Chemical reactivity</u>: Dibenzo(a,e)pyrene (DB(a,e)P) is oxidized by $Na_2Cr_2O_7$ in glacial acetic acid first to dibenzo(a,e)pyrene-8,14-quinone and then to 9,14-dioxo-9,14-dihydro-dibenz(a,c)anthracene carboxylic acid (Zinke & Zimmer, 1951; Ott, 1955). DB(a,e)P reacts with Br_2 or acetylchloride to give the mono substitution products 1-bromodibenzo(a,e)pyrene or 1-acetodibenzo(a,e)pyrene (Lang & Zander, 1965). Data on the reactive centre (K-region) are presented by Meyer & Bergmann (1969).

2. Use and Occurrence

(<u>a</u>) Analytical methods

Several chromatographic procedures for the separation of DB(a,e)P from other substances and for its spectroscopic determination have been published and are extensively reviewed by Sawicki (1964) and by Schaad (1970). They include column chromatography, used for detection in air (Dikun, 1967); thin-layer chromatography (Libičková et al., 1969; Dikun,

1967); gas chromatography, used for detection in cigarette smoke (Davis, 1969); gel chromatography (Edstrom & Petro, 1968); fluorescence spectroscopy (Dikun, 1967); and an electrophoretic separation method (Rothwell & Whitehead, 1967).

(b) Occurrence

Only one investigation on the occurrence of DB(a,e)P is known: Lyons (1959) detected the substance in petrol engine exhaust samples but made no quantitative determination.

3. Biological Data Relevant to the Evaluation of Carcinogenic Risk to Man

3.1 Carcinogenicity and related studies in animals

(a) Skin application

Mouse: Groups of 20 female Swiss albino Ha/ICR/Mil mice were painted thrice weekly for 12 months with either a 0.1% or a 0.05% solution of DB(a,e)P in dioxane. At the highest dose, nine out of 20 animals developed 12 papillomas and six carcinomas, whereas at the lowest dose 16/40 developed 16 papillomas and nine epitheliomas. 50% of the mice receiving the 0.05% solution had tumours at 15 months, whereas in a parallel experiment with benzo(a)pyrene at the same concentration tumours appeared in 50% of mice at six months. No tumours appeared among 20 controls given dioxane only (Hoffmann & Wynder, 1966).

(b) Subcutaneous and/or intramuscular administration

Mouse: Mice of the XVII Inc/Z strain of either sex received either three injections (at monthly intervals) or a single injection of 0.6 mg DB(a,e)P in olive oil. In the group receiving a total dose of 1.8 mg, 32/35 mice developed sarcomas within 142 days. In the group receiving 0.6 mg, 20/27 mice developed sarcomas within 220 days. No sex difference was observed (Lacassagne et al., 1963).

3.2 Other relevant biological data

None were available to the Working Group.

3.3 Observations in man

None were available to the Working Group.

4. Comments on Data Reported and Evaluation

4.1 Animal data

DB(a,e)P has produced tumours in mice following skin paintings and s.c. injection. In skin painting experiments, DB(a,e)P was less active than benzo(a)pyrene. It has not been tested by other routes in the mouse or in other species.

4.2 Human data

No case reports or epidemiological studies on the significance of DB(a,e)P exposure to man are available. The only reported occurrence of this substance was in the exhaust of internal combustion engines.

5. References

Beilsteins Handbuch der Organischen Chemie, 5, III, 2621

Clar, E. (1964) Polycyclic Hydrocarbons, Vol. 2, London, New York, Academic Press; Berlin, Göttingen, Heidelberg. Springer-Verlag, p. 145

Davis, H.J. (1969) Gas-chromatographic display of the polycyclic aromatic hydrocarbon fraction of cigarette smoke. Talanta, 16, 621

Demisch, R.R. & Wright, G.F. (1963) The distribution of polynuclear aromatic hydrocarbons between aqueous and non-aqueous phases. Canad. J. Biochem., 41, 1655

Dikun, P.P. (1967) Detection of polycyclic aromatic hydrocarbons in atmospheric contamination and other materials with quasi linear fluorescence spectra. Zh. Prikl. Spektrosk., 6, 202

Edstrom, T. & Petro, B.A. (1968) Gel permeation chromatographic studies of polynuclear aromatic hydrocarbon materials. J. polymer Sci. C, 21, 171

Hoffmann, D. & Wynder, E.L. (1966) Beitrag zur carcinogenen Wirkung von Dibenzopyrenen. Z. Krebsforsch., 68, 137

Lacassagne, A., Buu-Hoi, N.P., Zajdela, F. & Lavit-Lamy, D. (1963) Activité cancérogène élevée du 1,2,3,4-dibenzopyrène et 1,2,4,5-dibenzopyrène. C.R. Acad. Sci. (Paris), 256, 2728

Lang, K.F. & Zander, M. (1965) Zur Kenntnis des 1,2,4,5-Dibenzo-pyrens. Chem. Ber., 98, 597

Libičková, V., Stuchlik, M. & Krasnec, L. (1969) Chromatography of aromatic hydrocarbons on impregnated layers. J. Chromat., 45, 278

Lyons, M.J. (1959) Vehicular exhausts. Identification of further carcinogens of the polycyclic aromatic hydrocarbon class. Brit. J. Cancer, 13, 126

Meyer, A.Y. & Bergmann, E.D. (1969) Reactivity indices and carcinogenic activity of polynuclear aromatic hydrocarbons. In: Bergmann, E.D. & Pullman, B., eds., The Jerusalem Symposia on Quantum Chemistry and Biochemistry, Vol. 1, Physico-Chemical Mechanisms of Carcinogenesis, Jerusalem, The Israel Academy of Sciences and Humanities, p. 78

Ott, R. (1955) Synthese höher kondensierter Ringsysteme durch intermolekulare Dehydrierung verschiedener Moleküle unter Verknüpfung und Ringschluss. IX. Über das 1,2,4,5-Dibenzpyrenchinon, mit Bemerkungen über amphi- und o-Chinone. Mh. Chem., 86, 622

Rothwell, K. & Whitehead, J.K. (1967) A method for the isolation of polycyclic aromatic hydrocarbons from complex hydrocarbon mixtures. <u>Chem. and Ind.</u>, 784

Sawicki, E. (1964) The separation and analysis of polynuclear aromatic hydrocarbons present in the human environment. I-III. <u>Chemist-Analyst</u>, <u>53</u>, 24, 56, 88

Sawicki, E. (1969) Fluorescence analysis in air pollution research. <u>Talanta</u>, <u>16</u>, 1231

Sawicki, E., Hauser, T.R. & Stanley, T.W. (1960) Ultraviolet, visible and fluorescence spectral analysis of polynuclear hydrocarbons. <u>Int. J. air Pollut.</u>, <u>2</u>, 253

Schaad, R.E. (1970) Chromatographie (karzinogener) polycyclischer aromatischer Kohlenwasserstoffe. <u>Chromat. Rev.</u>, <u>13</u>, 61

Zinke, A. & Zimmer, W. (<u>1951</u>) Über die Bildung von Benzpyrenen aus Chrysenen. II. Über das 1,2,4,5-Dibenzpyren. <u>Mh. Chem.</u>, <u>82</u>, 348

DIBENZO(a,h)PYRENE*

1. Chemical and Physical Data

1.1 Synonyms

Chem. Abstr. No.: 189-64-0

Chem. Abstr. Name: Dibenzo(b,def)chrysene

1,2,6,7-Dibenzopyrene; 3,4,8,9-Dibenzopyrene; DB(a,h)P

1.2 Chemical formula and molecular weight

$C_{24}H_{14}$ Mol. wt: 302.38

1.3 Chemical and physical properties of the pure substance

(a) Description: Golden yellow plates from xylene or trichlorobenzene. General description in Beilsteins handbook, and in Clar (1964).

(b) Melting-point: 308°C, 310°C, 315°C

(c) Absorption spectroscopy: The ultra-violet absorption spectrum is described by Clar (1964); Van Duuren (1960); Schoental & Scott (1949), in petrol ether; and by Badger et al. (1965), who also give the fluorescence spectrum. Haigh & Mallion (1970) reported on the nuclear magnetic resonance spectrum.

---

*Considered by the Working Group in Lyon, December 1972.

(d) <u>Solubility and/or volatility</u>: The substance is soluble in H_2SO_4. The solution has a red colour, changing later into violet or blue.

(e) <u>Chemical reactivity</u>: Data on reactive centres in the molecule (K-region) are given by Sung (1967) and by Meyer & Bergmann (1969). Pullman (1964) reported on the electron density. Binding lengths are indicated by Vasudevan & Laidlaw (1969). The mono- or dinitro derivative is formed by nitration (Ioffe & Efross, 1946).

2. Use and Occurrence

(a) <u>Analytical methods</u>

Several chromatographic procedures for the separation of dibenzo(a,h)pyrene (DB(a,h)P) from other substances are published. They include paper chromatography (Stuchlík et al., 1967), used for detection in food (Masuda et al., 1966); thin-layer chromatography (Hood & Winefordner, 1968), used for detection in air (Matsushita et al., 1970); gas chromatography, used for detection in cigarette smoke (Carugno & Rossi, 1967); and gel chromatography, used for detection in air (Klimisch & Reese, 1972). Subsequent determination by fluorescence spectroscopy (Matsushita et al., 1970) or by low-temperature fluorescence (Hood & Winefordner, 1968) and an electrophoretic separation method (Rothwell & Whitehead, 1967) are also described.

(b) <u>Occurrence</u>

In comparison with other polycyclic aromatic hydrocarbons, only few investigations on the occurrence of DB(a,h)P have been made.

The Surgeon General's Report (1962) indicated that DB(a,h)P may be found in air pollutants or engine exhaust.

According to Lyons & Johnston (1957) minute amounts of DB(a,h)P are present in the neutral fraction of cigarette tar.

Badger et al. (1964, 1965, 1966) indicated that DB(a,h)P is formed by the pyrolysis of anthracene at 700-850°C, of the tobacco constituents dotriacontane or stigmasterol at 700°C and of isoprene at 700°C.

Buu-Hoï (1958) isolated small amounts in various samples of coal-tar pitch.

3. Biological Data Relevant to the Evaluation of Carcinogenic Risk to Man

3.1 Carcinogenicity and related studies in animals

(a) Skin application

Mouse: The carcinogenic action of DB(a,h)P was studied by Kleinenberg (1939) in 74 young P-B mice by means of skin painting. A drop of a saturated solution of the compound in benzene (0.15-0.18%) was applied every other day to 50 male mice 86 times. Epitheliomata were observed in 32 mice (65%) in this group; 49 animals were alive at three-and-a-half months when the first tumour appeared. The other group of 14 male and 10 female mice received the same dose every third day 55 times. Eleven epitheliomata developed, 23 animals being alive at three-and-a-half months. The animals were kept for at least four-and-a-half months. An increase in the incidence of distant tumours, adenomata of the sebaceous glands and of the lungs was reported in both sexes in this group, the incidences being 45% and 34%, respectively. The spontaneous incidences of these tumours in control animals of this strain were reported to be 0.15-1% for sebaceous adenomas and 5-8.5% for lung adenomas.

Badger et al. (1940) applied a 0.3% solution in benzene twice weekly to the skin of 30 stock mice. The experiment lasted for 350 days, and 10 carcinomas were recorded.

Hoffmann & Wynder (1966) painted two groups of 20 female Ha/ICR/Mil (Swiss Albino) mice thrice weekly for 12 months with a 0.1% or 0.05% solution of DB(a,h)P in dioxane. In the first group 15 animals developed 58 papillomas and 20 epitheliomas, and in the second group 16 animals developed 44 papillomas and 15 epitheliomas. The mean latent periods were 196 and 224 days, respectively. The control group of 20 animals given dioxane alone did not develop tumours. The time at which 50% of the mice receiving the 0.05% solution had tumours was nine months, whereas in a parallel experiment with benzo(a)pyrene at the same concentration it was six months.

(b) Subcutaneous and/or intramuscular administration

Mouse: Kleinenberg (1938) injected 20 white mice subcutaneously with 6 mg DB(a,h)P dissolved in pure olive oil. Malignant tumours developed at the injection site in 17 animals surviving after three-and-a-half months. The experiment lasted for nine-and-a-half months, by which time all animals had died.

Mice of XVII strain were given three injections at monthly intervals of 0.6 mg DB(a,h)P in 0.2 ml olive oil. A total of 34 sarcomas in 35 males and one sarcoma in 10 females were induced. The mean latent periods were 111 and 128 days, respectively (Lacassagne et al., 1958).

Rat: Voronjansky et al. (1939) reported the occurrence of two tumours in four rats dying after seven to eight months following i.m. administration of 0.5-1.0 mg of DB(a,h)P in sunflower-seed oil. The duration of the experiment was at least eight months. In another study, six females were injected with a single dose of 0.5 mg DB(a,h)P in rabbit fat, and two sarcomas appeared at five-and-a-half and eight months (Pisareva et al., 1940).

3.2 Other relevant biological data

No data were available to the Working Group.

3.3 Observations in man

No data were available to the Working Group.

4. Comments on Data Reported and Evaluation

4.1 Animal data

Carcinogenic effects of DB(a,h)P were demonstrated following repeated skin painting in mice and injections in mice and rats. In the skin painting experiment, it was less active than benzo(a)pyrene. It has not been tested by other routes or in other species.

4.2 Human data

No case reports or epidemiological studies on the significance of DB(a,h)P exposure to man are available. However, coal-tar and other materials which are known to be carcinogenic to man may contain DB(a,h)P. The substance has also been detected in other environmental situations. The possible contribution of polycyclic aromatic hydrocarbons from some environmental sources to the overall carcinogenic risk to man is discussed in the preamble.

5. References

Badger, G.M., Cook, J.W., Hewett, C.L., Kennaway, E.L., Kennaway, N.M., Martin, R.H. & Robinson, A.M. (1940) The production of cancer by pure hydrocarbons. V. Proc. roy. Soc. London B, 129, 439

Badger, G.M., Donnelly, J.K. & Spotswood, T.M. (1964) Formation of aromatic hydrocarbons at high temperatures. XIII. Pyrolysis of anthracene. Aust. J. Chem., 17, 1147

Badger, G.M., Donnelly, J.K. & Spotswood, T.M. (1965) The formation of aromatic hydrocarbons at high temperatures. XXIV. The pyrolysis of some tobacco constituents. Aust. J. Chem., 18, 1249

Badger, G.M., Donnelly, J.K. & Spotswood, T.M. (1966) Formation of aromatic hydrocarbons at high temperatures. XXVII. The pyrolysis of isoprene. Aust. J. Chem., 19, 1023

Beilsteins Handbuch der Organischen Chemie, 5, III, 2619

Buu-Hoï, N.P. (1958) Presence of 3,4,8,9-dibenzpyrene in coal-tar. Nature (Lond.), 182, 1158

Carugno, N. & Rossi, S. (1967) Evaluation of polynuclear hydrocarbons in cigarette smoke by glass capillary columns. J. gas Chromat., 5, 103

Clar, E. (1964) Polycyclic Hydrocarbons, Vol. 2, London, New York, Academic Press; Berlin, Göttingen, Heidelberg, Springer-Verlag, p. 151

Haigh, C.W. & Mallion, R.B. (1970) Proton magnetic resonance of planar condensed benzenoid hydrocarbons. Molec. Phys. 18, 767

Hoffmann, D. & Wynder, E.L. (1966) Beitrag zur carcinogenen Wirkung von Dibenzopyrenen. Z. Krebsforsch., 68, 137

Hood, L.V.S. & Winefordner, J.D. (1968) Thin-layer separation and low-temperature luminescence measurement of mixtures of carcinogens. Analyt. Chim. Acta, 42, 199

Ioffe, I.S. & Efross, L.S. (1946) Nitro and amino derivatives of dibenzopyrene. J. gen. Chem. (USSR), 16, 111

Kleinenberg, H.E. (1938) On the blastogenic effect of 3,4,8,9-dibenzpyrene and some of its derivatives. I. Tumours caused by subcutaneous injection of dibenzpyrene. Arh. Biol. Nauk., 51, 127

Kleinenberg, H.E. (1939) Investigations on the blastomogenic effect of 3,4,8,9-dibenzpyrene and some of its derivatives. II. Tumours called forth by painting the skin with dibenzpyrene. Arh. Biol. Nauk., 56, 39

Klimisch, H.J. & Reese, D. (1972) Das gelchromatographische Trennverhalten von Polystyrolgel für Kohlenwasserstoffe, Amine and Phenole. Präparative Fraktionierung von Cigarettenrauchkondensat für biologische Versuche. J. Chromat., 67, 299

Lacassagne, A., Buu-Hoï, N.P. & Zajdela, F. (1958) Relation entre structure moléculaire et activité cancérogène dans trois séries d'hydrocarbures aromatiques hexacycliques. C.R. Acad. Sci. (Paris), 246, 1477

Lyons, M.J. & Johnston, H. (1957) Chemical investigation of the neutral fraction of cigarette smoke tar. Brit. J. Cancer, 11, 554

Matsushita, H., Esumi, Y. & Yamada, K. (1970) Identification of polynuclear hydrocarbons in air pollutants. Bunseki Kagaku, 19, 951

Meyer, A.Y. & Bergmann, E.D. (1969) Reactivity indices and carcinogenic activity of polynuclear aromatic hydrocarbons. In: Bergmann, E.D. & Pullman, B., eds., The Jerusalem Symposia on Quantum Chemistry and Biochemistry, Vol. 1, Physico-Chemical Mechanisms of Carcinogenesis, Jerusalem, The Israel Academy of Sciences and Humanities, p. 78

Pisareva, T.A., Ber, L.S. & Sorin, J.E. (1940) Activity of cancerogenic compounds of Soviet production. Tr. Perv. Syezda Onkol., 31

Pullman, B. (1964) Electronic aspects of the interactions between the carcinogens and possible cellular sites of their activity. J. cell. comp. Physiol., 64, Suppl. 1, 91

Rothwell, K. & Whitehead, J.K. (1967) Isolation of polycyclic aromatic hydrocarbons from complex hydrocarbon mixtures. Chem. and Ind., 784

Schoental, R. & Scott, E.J.Y. (1949) Fluorescence spectra of polycyclic aromatic hydrocarbons in solution. J. chem. Soc., 1683

Stuchlík, M., Krasnec, Ľ. & Csiba, I. (1967) The use of solubilizing agents in partition paper chromatography. III. The separation of aromatic hydrocarbons in the mobile phase. J. Chromat., 30, 543

Sung, S. (1967) Sur l'existence éventuelle d'une corrélation plus générale entre le pouvoir cancérogène d'une substance et une de ses propriétés moléculaires. C.R. Acad. Sci. (Paris), Ser. D, 264, 189

Surgeon General's Report (1962) Motor vehicles, air pollution and health, Washington, D.C., Government Printing Office (Public Health Service Publication No. 489)

Van Duuren, B.L. (1960) The fluorescence spectra of aromatic hydrocarbons and heterocyclic aromatic compounds. Analyt. Chem., 32, 1436

Vasudevan, K. & Laidlaw, W.G. (1969) Self-consistent iterative technique for bond length calculations. II. Tables of bond length data. Coll. Cs. chem. Commun., 34, 361

Voronjansky, G.S., Pisareva, T.A. & Sorin, J.E. (1939) The histological picture of the tumours caused by the synthetic cancerogenic hydrocarbons of Soviet make (dibenzepyrene and hydrodibenzepyrene). Arh. Biol. Nauk, 55, 89

DIBENZO(a,i)PYRENE[*]

1. Chemical and Physical Data

1.1 Synonyms

Chem. Abstr. No.: 189-55-9

Chem. Abstr. Name: Benzo(r,s,t)pentaphene

3,4,9,10-Dibenzpyrene; 1,2,7,8-Dibenzopyrene; DB(a,i)P

1.2 Chemical formula and molecular weight

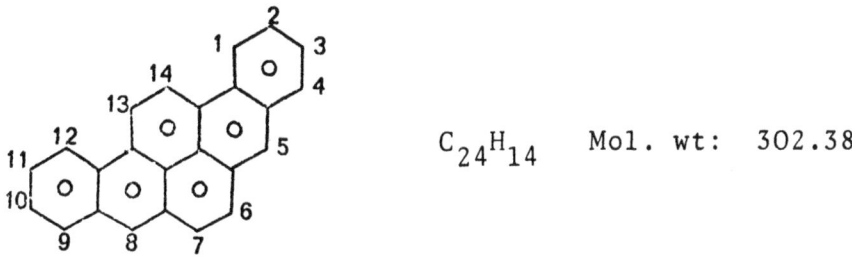

$C_{24}H_{14}$ Mol. wt: 302.38

1.3 Chemical and physical properties of the pure substance

(a) *Description*: Greenish-yellow needles, prisms or lamellae. General description in Beilsteins handbook, and in Clar (1964).

(b) *Melting-point*: 280°C (from xylene); 281.5-282°C (from benzene)

(c) *Absorption spectroscopy*: Clar (1964) gives the ultra-violet absorption spectrum in benzene, and Muel et al. (1957) the fluorescence spectrum in cyclohexane. Ultra-violet and fluorescence spectra are also mentioned by Badger et al. (1965).

---

[*] Considered by the Working Group in Lyon, December 1972.

(d) _Solubility and/or volatility_: One part of dibenzo(a,i)pyrene (DB(a,i)P) is soluble in 500 parts of boiling glacial acetic acid and in 200 parts of boiling benzene. The solution has a yellow colour and a blue fluorescence. Concentrated H_2SO_4 solutions are blue with red fluorescence. It is almost insoluble in alcohol and ether. DB(a,i)P can be sublimed unchanged.

(e) _Chemical reactivity_: DB(a,i)P is attacked by nitric acid and by other reagents, mainly at the 5 and 8 positions. With $Pb(OAc)_4$, it is oxidized to a dihydric alcohol, and to quinones with CrO_3 or SeO_2 (Ünseren & Fieser, 1962). In sulphuric acid it is slowly oxidized to quinone.

2. Use and Occurrence

(a) Analytical methods

Several chromatographic procedures for the separation of DB(a,i)P from other substances have been published and are reviewed by Schaad (1970). They include paper chromatography (Stuchlík et al., 1967; Monkman & Porro, 1960); thin-layer chromatography (White & Howard, 1967; Hood & Winefordner, 1968); and gas chromatography, used for detection in tobacco smoke (Chortyk et al., 1965). Subsequent determination by fluorescence spectroscopy (Monkman & Porro, 1960) or low-temperature spectroscopy (Hood & Winefordner, 1968) and an electrophoretic separation method (Rothwell & Whitehead, 1967) are described. References to analytical methods used for detection in various other media, such as air and cigarette smoke, can be found in the section on "Occurrence".

(b) Occurrence

In comparison with other polycyclic hydrocarbons, few investigations of the occurrence of DB(a,i)P have been made.

Hoffmann & Wynder (1962) found traces of DB(a,i)P in automobile exhaust gas.

Bonnet & Neukomm (1956) and Wynder & Wright (1957) indicate that cigarette smoke contains traces of DB(a,i)P. According to the Surgeon General's Report (1964), 0.002-1 µg DB(a,i)P was present in the smoke from 100 cigarettes. Müller et al. (1967) found 0.17 µg DB(a,i)P in the smoke from 100 cigarettes, and 0.27 µg DB(a,i)P in 100 g of smoked tobacco.

Schoental (1957) showed that DB(a,i)P is present in coal-tar.

3. Biological Data Relevant to the Evaluation of Carcinogenic Risk to Man

3.1 Carcinogenicity and related studies in animals

(a) Skin application

Mouse: Lacassagne et al. (1958) observed 21 papillomas and eight epitheliomas on the skin of 23 mice (XVII strain) painted twice weekly with a saturated solution of DB(a,i)P in peanut oil after a latent period of 83 days. Pai & Ranadive (1965) applied a saturated solution of DB(a,i)P in benzene to the skin of 12 mice and found that four mice developed epidermoid carcinoma after 11 months. Hoffmann & Wynder (1966) painted groups of 20 female Swiss albino Ha/ICR/Mil mice thrice weekly for 12 months with solutions in dioxane; 16

animals developed 15 epitheliomas and 29 papillomas after treatment with a 0.1% solution, and 16 animals developed 13 epitheliomas and 28 papillomas after treatment with a 0.05% solution. The time at which 50% of the mice treated with the 0.05% solution had tumours was 11 months, whereas in a parallel experiment with the same concentration of benzo(a)pyrene it was six months. No tumours appeared among 20 controls given dioxane only.

(b) Subcutaneous and/or intramuscular administration

Mouse: Lacassagne et al. (1957) injected 0.6 mg DB(a,i)P in peanut oil three times at monthly intervals to 11 mice (XVII strain). All animals developed sarcomas at the site of injection beginning at the 42nd day after injection. Following three s.c. applications of 0.6 mg DB(a,i)P Lacassagne et al. (1958) observed 33 sarcomas in 35 mice (XVII strain). Waravdekar & Ranadive (1958) produced sarcomas in all of 16 mice (a cross of two inbred strains: XVII and C57BL) within three months following single s.c. injections of 2 mg DB(a,i)P suspended in 0.2 ml propylene glycol. Schoental (1959) gave six albino mice single s.c. injections of a suspension of 2 mg DB(a,i)P in 0.1 ml medicinal paraffin oil, and six mice 4 mg in 0.2 ml oil. All animals developed sarcomas at the site of injection, half of them within two-and-a-half months.

Homburger & Treger (1960) gave single s.c. injections into the groins of over 10 000 C57 mice of 0.5 mg DB(a,i)P in tricaprylin and produced sarcomas at the site of injection in 50% of mice in 14 weeks and in 98% of mice in 24 weeks. High tumour yields after s.c. injections have been described elsewhere (Biedler, 1962; Pai & Ranadive, 1965). Epstein et al. (1967) observed 125 fibrosarcomas and two local carcinomas in 138 ICR/Ha Swiss mice which survived the treatment (a single injection of 100 mg DB(a,i)P in 0.2 ml tricaprylin) and were followed for 10 weeks. Old et al. (1962) injected 50 or 100 µg DB(a,i)P in sesame oil to groups of eight to 25 mice of both sexes of different strains of mice and observed them for eight months. Incidences of 91-100% sarcomas were obtained in BALB/c and C3H mice and their hybrids, while in I mice incidences were slightly lower.

Hamster: Single injections of 250, 500, 1000 or 2000 µg DB(a,i)P in tricaprylin induced sarcomas in 5/9, 9/10, 10/10 and 6/6 hamsters in 17-27 weeks (Wodinsky et al., 1964).

(c) Other experimental systems

Transfer of injection sites: Homburger & Baker (1969) gave C57BL/6 J mice single s.c. injections of 25 µg DB(a,i)P in 0.1 ml of tricaprylin. After seven weeks the injection sites were removed, minced in Ringer's solution and injected s.c. into new hosts. This method shortened the latent period. Fifty animals used as positive control showed 100% tumour incidence in 23 weeks. Homburger & Treger (1967, 1970) demonstrated that transfer of sites of injection of DB(a,i)P (25-500 µg) accelerates tumour growth in the second recipient. The latent period was shortened by up to five weeks.

3.2 Other relevant biological data

(a) Animals: Kelley (1970) injected C57/BL/6 Jax mice s.c. with 500 µg ^{14}C-labelled DB(a,i)P in peanut oil. The distribution of radioactivity between injection sites and organs was determined. This experiment demonstrated that 85% of the carcinogen is removed from the injection site and that the removal was nearly complete in 10 weeks.

3.3 Observations in man

No data were available to the Working Group.

4. Comments on Data Reported and Evaluation

4.1 Animal data

S.c. injections of DB(a,i)P resulted in the rapid appearance of local sarcomas in the hamster and the mouse. The smallest single dose which produced sarcomas in mice was 50 µg. Repeated skin application in mice was also effective, but DB(a,i)P was less active than benzo(a)pyrene. It has not been tested by other routes or in other species.

4.2 Human data

No case reports or epidemiological studies on the significance of DB(a,i)P exposure to man are available. However, coal-tar and other materials which are known to be carcinogenic to man may contain DB(a,i)P. The substance has also been detected in other environmental situations. The possible contribution of polycyclic aromatic hydrocarbons from some environmental sources to the overall carcinogenic risk to man is discussed in the preamble.

5. References

Badger, G.M., Donnelly, J.K. & Spotswood, T.M. (1965) The formation of aromatic hydrocarbons at high temperatures. XXIV. The pyrolysis of some tobacco constituents. Aust. J. Chem., 18, 1249

Beilsteins Handbuch der Organischen Chemie, 5, II, 688; 5, III, 2620

Biedler, J.L. (1962) Chromosomal patterns in chemically-induced tumors in mice. Proc. amer. Ass. Cancer Res., 3, 304

Bonnet, J. & Neukomm, S. (1956) Sur la composition chimique de la fumée du tabac. I. Analyse de la fraction neutre. Helv. chim. Acta, 39, 1724

Chortyk, O.T., Schlotzhauer, W.S. & Stedmann, R.L. (1965) Lithium chloride as a gas-chromatographic substrate for polynuclear aromatic hydrocarbons. J. gas Chromat., 3, 394

Clar, E. (1964) Polycyclic Hydrocarbons, Vol. 2, London, New York, Academic Press; Berlin, Göttingen, Heidelberg, Springer-Verlag, p. 153

Epstein, S.S., Joshi, S., Andrea, J., Forsyth, J. & Mantel, N. (1967) The null effect of antioxidants on the carcinogenicity of 3,4,9,10-dibenzpyrene to mice. Life Sci., 6, 225

Hoffmann, D. & Wynder, E.L. (1962) Analytical and biological studies on gasoline engine exhaust. Nat. Cancer Inst. Monogr., 9, 91

Hoffmann, D. & Wynder, E.L. (1966) Beitrag zur carcinogenen Wirkung von Dibenzopyrenen. Z. Krebsforsch., 68, 137

Homburger, F. & Baker, J.R. (1969) Accelerated carcinogen testing. Progr. exp. tumor Res. (Basel), 11, 384

Homburger, F. & Treger, A. (1960) Modifying factors in carcinogenesis. Progr. exp. tumor Res. (Basel), 1, 311

Homburger, F. & Treger, A. (1967) Acceleration of growth of chemically induced tumors by use of transplantation technic. Cancer Res., 27, 1205

Homburger, F. & Treger, A. (1970) Transplantation technique for acceleration of carcinogenesis by benz(a)anthracene or 3,4,9,10-dibenzpyrene (benzo(rst)pentaphene). J. nat. Cancer Inst., 44, 357

Hood, L.V. & Winefordner, J.D. (1968) Thin-layer separation and low-temperature measurement of mixtures of carcinogens. Analyt. Chim. Acta, 42, 199

Kelley, T.F. (1970) Fate of subcutaneously injected benzo(rst)pentaphene in C57BL/6 mice. Proc. Soc. exp. Biol. (N.Y.), 133, 1402

Lacassagne, A., Zajdela, F., Buu-Hoï, N.P. & Chalvet, H. (1957) Sur l'activité cancérogène du 3,4,9,10-dibenzopyrène et de quelques-uns de ses dérivés. C.R. Acad. Sci. (Paris), 244, 273

Lacassagne, A., Buu-Hoï, N.P. & Zajdela, F. (1958) Relation entre structure moléculaire et activité cancérogène dans trois séries d'hydrocarbures aromatiques hexacycliques. C.R. Acad. Sci. (Paris), 246, 1477

Monkman, J.L. & Porro, T.J. (1960) Identification of polycyclic aromatic hydrocarbons by ultra-violet fluorescence. In: Proceedings of the 6th Symposium on Instrumental Methods of Analysis, Montreal, Pittsburgh, Instrument Society of America, p. D4

Muel, B., Hubert-Habart, M. & Buu-Hoï, N.P. (1957) Etude du dibenzo,3,4,9,10-pyrene: spectre de fluorescence et séparation chromatographique du benzo-3,4-pyrene. J. Chim. phys., 54, 483

Müller, R., Moldenhauer, W. & Schlemmer, P. (1967) Erfahrungen bei der quantitativen Bestimmung von polyzyklischen Kohlenwasserstoffen im Tabakrauch. Ber. Inst. Tabakforsch. (Dresden), 14, 159

Old, L.J., Boyse, E.A., Clarke, D.A. & Carswell, E.A. (1962) Antigenic properties of chemically induced tumours. II. Antigens of tumor cells. Ann. N.Y. Acad. Sci., 101, 80

Pai, S.R. & Ranadive, K.J. (1965) Biological testing of analogues of 3,4-benzpyrene. Indian J. med. Res., 53, 638

Rothwell, K. & Whitehead, J.K. (1967) Isolation of polycyclic aromatic hydrocarbons from complex hydrocarbon mixtures. Chem. and Ind., 784

Schaad, R.E. (1970) Chromatographie (karzinogener) polycyclischer aromatischer Kohlenwasserstoffe. Chromat. Rev., 13, 61

Schoental, R. (1957) Isolation of 3,4,9,10-dibenzopyrene from coal-tar. Nature (Lond.), 180, 606

Schoental, R. (1959) Carcinogenic activity of 3,4,9,10-dibenzopyrene. Un. int. Cancr. Acta, 15, 216

Stuchlík, M., Krasnec, L. & Csiba, T. (1967) The use of solubilizing agents in partition paper chromatography. III. The separation of aromatic hydrocarbons by solubilizers in mobile phase. J. Chromat., 30, 534

Surgeon General's Report (1964) Smoking and health, Washington, D.C., Government Printing Office (Public Health Service Publication No. 1103)

Ünseren, E. & Fieser, F.L. (1962) Investigation of the metabolism of 3,4,9,10-dibenzpyrene. J. org. Chem., 27, 1386

Waravdekar, S.S. & Ranadive, K.J. (1958) Biologic testing of 3,4,9,10-dibenz-pyrene. J. nat. Cancer Inst., 21, 1151

White, R.H. & Howard, J.W. (1967) Thin-layer chromatography of polycyclic aromatic hydrocarbons. J. Chromat., 29, 108

Wodinsky, I., Helinsky, A. & Kensler, C.J. (1964) Susceptibility of Syrian hamsters to induction of fibrosarcomas with a single injection of 3,4,9,10-dibenzpyrene. Nature (Lond.), 203, 308

Wynder, E.L. & Wright, G. (1957) Study of tobacco carcinogenesis. I. Primary fractions. Cancer, 10, 255

DIBENZO(a,l)PYRENE*

1. Chemical and Physical Data

1.1 Synonyms

Chem. Abstr. No.: 191-30-0

Chem. Abstr. Name: Dibenzo(def,p)chrysene

1,2,9,10-Dibenzopyrene; 1,2,3,4-Dibenzopyrene; DB(a,l)P

1.2 Chemical formula and molecular weight

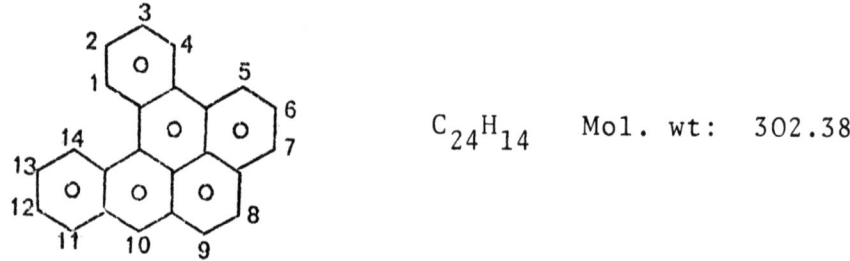

$C_{24}H_{14}$ Mol. wt: 302.38

1.3 Chemical and physical properties of the pure substance

(a) Description: Pale yellow plates from ethanol, or pale yellow plates from ethanol/benzene. The compound described in Beilsteins handbook and in Clar (1964) as dibenzo(a,l)pyrene is, according to Lavit-Lamy & Buu-Hoï (1966), dibenzo(a,e)fluoranthene (melting-point 224-232°C). Therefore, it may be that some, probably all, investigations former to 1966 concerning dibenzo(a,l)pyrene were carried out with dibenzo(a,e)fluoranthene.

(b) Melting-point: 162-164°C (Vingiello et al., 1966; Carruthers, 1966, 1967).

---

* Considered by the Working Group in Lyon, December 1972.

(c) <u>Absorption spectroscopy</u>: Carruthers (1966, 1967) describes the ultra-violet absorption spectrum in ethanolic solution.

(d) <u>Identity and purity test</u>: The 1,3,5-trinitrobenzene complex forms crimson needles (melting-point 205-206°C).

(e) <u>Solubility and/or volatility</u>: In concentrated sulphuric acid, the hydrocarbon gives a transient deep blue colour, rapidly changing to crimson. The solubilization in water by purines and pyrimidines is described by Caillet & Pullman (1968).

(f) <u>Chemical reactivity</u>: Data on reactive centres in the molecule (K-region) are given by Sung (1967).

2. Use and Occurrence

(a) <u>Analytical methods</u>

Several chromatographic procedures for the separation of dibenzo(a,l)pyrene (DB(a,l)P) from other substances have been published. They include paper chromatography (Stuchlík et al., 1967; Maly, 1969); thin-layer chromatography (Libičková et al., 1969; Hood & Winefordner, 1968), used for detection in air (Siburu et al., 1967); gas chromatography (Savino, 1968), used for detection in cigarette smoke (Davis, 1969); and an electrophoretic separation method (Rothwell & Whitehead, 1967).

(b) <u>Occurrence</u>

It is probable that all investigations prior to 1966 reporting the occurrence of dibenzo(a,l)pyrene in different media were in fact detecting dibenzo(a,e)fluoranthrene (see section 1.3 of this monograph), therefore no data on its occurrence are available to the Working Group.

3. Biological Data Relevant to the Evaluation of Carcinogenic Risk to Man

3.1 Carcinogenicity and related studies in animals[1]

(a) <u>Subcutaneous and/or intramuscular administration</u>

<u>Mouse</u>: Lacassagne et al. (1968) gave two subcutaneous injections of 0.6 mg DB(a,l)P in 0.2 ml olive oil at one month intervals to 12 mice of each sex of strain XVII nc/ZE. After two months a third injection was given to a few mice which had not developed a strong fibrous reaction at the site of injection. All animals developed sarcomas at the injection site. The mean latent periods were 130 days for males and 113 days for females.

3.2 Other relevant biological data

None were available to the Working Group.

3.3 Observations in man

No data were available to the Working Group.

4. Comments on Data Reported and Evaluation

4.1 Animal data

Because of an error in identification, early experiments supposedly made with DB(a,l)P did not in fact deal with this compound. In the only study actually carried out with DB(a,l)P, sarcomas were induced in all animals following subcutaneous administration to mice. It has not been tested by other routes in mice or in other species.

---

[1] Only experiments carried out after 1966 have been considered.

4.2 Human data

No case reports or epidemiological studies on the significance of DB(a,l)P exposure to man are available. It is likely that it occurs in the environment, but the data available cannot be interpreted because of the identification problem mentioned above.

5. References

Beilsteins Handbuch der Organischen Chemie, 5, III, 2620

Caillet, J. & Pullman, B. (1968) Solubilization of aromatic carcinogens by purines and pyrimidines. In: Pullman, B., ed., Molecular Associations in Biology, New York, Academic Press, p. 217

Carruthers, W. (1966) Synthesis of dibenzo(a,l)pyrene. Chem. Commun., 548

Carruthers, W. (1967) Photocyclisation of some stilbene analogs. Synthesis of dibenzo(a,l)pyrene. J. chem. Soc. C, 1525

Clar, E. (1964) Polycyclic Hydrocarbons, Vol. 2, London, New York, Academic Press; Berlin, Göttingen, Heidelberg, Springer-Verlag, p. 141

Davis, H.J. (1969) Gas-chromatographic display of the polycyclic aromatic hydrocarbon fraction of cigarette smoke. Talanta, 16, 621

Hood, L.V.S. & Winefordner, J.D. (1968) Thin-layer separation and low-temperature luminescence measurement of mixtures of carcinogens. Analyt. Chim. Acta, 42, 199

Lacassagne, A., Buu-Hoï, N.P., Zajdela, F. & Vingiello, F.A. (1968) The true dibenzo(a,l)pyrene, a new potent carcinogen. Naturwissenschaften, 55, 43

Lavit-Lamy, D. & Buu-Hoï, N.P. (1966) The true nature of "dibenzo(a,l)pyrene" and its known derivatives. Chem. Commun., 92

Libičková, V., Stuchlík, M. & Krasnec, Ľ. (1969) Chromatography of aromatic hydrocarbons on impregnated layers. J. Chromat., 45, 278

Maly, E. (1969) Paper chromatography of tar polycyclic hydrocarbons. A correction of previous results. J. Chromat., 40, 190

Rothwell, K. & Whitehead, J.K. (1967) Isolation of polycyclic aromatic hydrocarbons from complex hydrocarbon mixtures. Chem. and Ind., 784

Savino, A. (1968) Determinazione per via gas cromatografica degli idrocarburi aromatici policiclici. Riv. ital. Igiene, 28, 56

Siburu, J.R., Catalina, R.L. & Singerman, A. (1967) Hidrocarburos aromaticos policiclicos y arsenico en la atmosfera de la ciudad de Buenos Aires. Rev. Asoc. bioquim. Argent., 32, 66

Stuchlík, M., Krasnec, Ľ. & Csiba, I. (1967) The use of solubilizing agents in partition paper chromatography. III. The separation of aromatic hydrocarbons in the mobile phase. J. Chromat., 30, 543

Sung, S. (1967) Sur l'existence éventuelle d'une corrélation plus générale entre le pouvoir cancérogène d'une substance et une de ses propriétés moléculaires. C.R. Acad. Sci. (Paris), Ser. D, 264, 189

Vingiello, F.A., Yanez, J. & Greenwood, E.J. (1966) The synthesis of dibenzo(a,l)pyrene. Chem. Commun., 375

INDENO(1,2,3-cd)PYRENE*

1. Chemical and Physical Data

1.1 Synonyms

Chem. Abstr. No.: 193-39-5

2,3-o-Phenylenepyrene; IP

1.2 Chemical formula and molecular weight

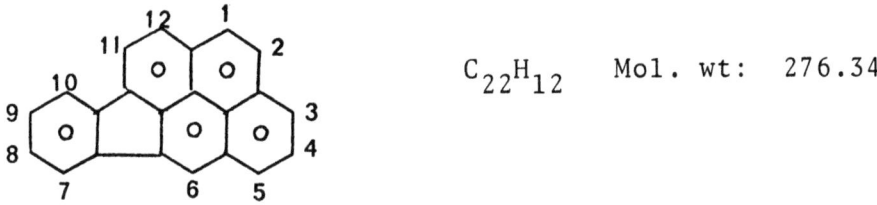

$C_{22}H_{12}$ Mol. wt: 276.34

1.3 Chemical and physical properties of the pure substance

(a) Description: Yellow plates or needles from light petroleum. General description in Clar (1964).

(b) Melting-point: 162.5-164°C

(c) Absorption spectroscopy: The ultra-violet absorption spectrum of the substance was described by Clar (1964); Hoffmann & Wynder (1962a), in cyclohexane; Badger et al. (1965); Lang & Buffleb (1957); Lang et al. (1959); and Sawicki et al. (1960), in pentane. Sawicki et al. (1960) also reported on the fluorescence maximum and on the relative molar extinction of the compound.

(d) Identity and purity test: The picrate decomposes at 150-180°C.

---

* Considered by the Working Group in Lyon, December 1972.

(e) *Solubility and/or volatility*: Solutions show a greenish yellow fluorescence.

2. Use and Occurrence

(a) *Analytical methods*

Several chromatographic procedures for the separation of indeno(1,2,3-cd)pyrene (IP) from other substances and for its subsequent determination by absorption or fluorescence spectroscopy have been published. They include paper chromatography; column chromatography, used for detection in soot (Chakraborty & Long, 1967); thin-layer chromatography, used for detection in air (Dikun, 1967; Matsushita et al., 1970); gas-chromatography (Chakraborty & Long, 1967); ultra-violet absorption spectroscopy (Chakraborty & Long, 1967); and fluorescence spectroscopy (Dikun, 1967; Matsushita et al., 1970). References to analytical methods used for detection in various other media such as air, water, food, etc. can be found in the section on "Occurrence".

(b) *Occurrence*

Exhaust: Hoffmann & Wynder (1962a,b) isolated 82 mg/kg of exhaust tar from first run gasoline engine exhaust, and 5.7 µg/minute run from automobile exhaust. In diesel engine exhaust, up to 11 $µg/m^3$ were found (Reckner et al., 1965).

Air: Concentrations ranging from 135-457 mg/kg IP were found in tar samples in the Detroit area (Colucci & Begeman, 1965); in road dust 8-61 mg/kg were found, and in dust from air 0.96 mg/kg (Borneff & Kunte, 1965).

Cigarette smoke: In the smoke condensate of 100 cigarettes concentrations ranged from 0.4 µg (Scassellati-Sforzolini et al., 1967; Wynder & Hoffmann, 1963) to 2 µg (Ayres & Thornton, 1965).

Pyrolysis: IP is formed on pyrolysis of the tobacco constituents dotriacontane or stigmasterol at 700°C (Badger et al., 1965), and of benzene and pyrene at 700°C (Lang & Buffleb, 1957).

Occupational exposure: An average value of 14.7 mg/kg was isolated from soot samples (Fischer, 1970). Lang et al. (1959) detected IP in coal-tar, and Wallcave et al. (1971) determined 7300-9300 mg/kg in coal-tar pitch and up to 1 mg/kg in petroleum asphalts.

Soil and water: Borneff & Fischer (1962) detected IP in soil samples of forest areas of Darmstadt, and Borneff & Fischer (1963) found 0.6 and 0.5 mg/kg in the muddy deposits of Lake Constance and of the Rhine river. In drinking-water, concentrations ranged from 0.1-12.6 µg/m^3 (Borneff & Kunte, 1964, 1969). In river and lake water a wide range of concentrations (17-4980 µg/m^3) has been found, depending on the kind of water tested (whether it contained industrial effluents or bituminous contamination) (Borneff & Kunte, 1965); while in surface water, concentrations ranged from 1.4-123 µg/m^3 (Borneff & Kunte, 1964). As much as 15 000 µg/m^3 have been found in sewage water (from households, industry and roads) (Borneff & Kunte, 1967).

Food: Fresh sausages contained 0.3 µg/kg, and charcoal broiling brought the content up to 9 µg/kg (Fábián, 1968b). In coconut oil, olive oil, plant cooking fat and plant oil, 0.9-1.6 µg/kg have been found

(Borneff & Fábián, 1966; Fábián, 1968a). Fábián (1968, 1969) detected concentrations of 0.2-5.5 µg/kg in margarine, the IP content being reduced considerably by treatment with activated charcoal and steam. The IP content of oil decreased slightly with frying (Fritz, 1968b), and that of fat with controlled laboratory heating (Borneff & Fábián, 1966). In normally roasted coffee no IP was found, but up to 0.8 µg/kg could be detected in extremely black coffee and up to 5.9 µg/kg in malt coffee, substitute coffee and soluble coffee powder (Fritz, 1968a, 1969).

Other material: IP is present in the leaves of various kinds of trees (26-234 µg/kg) and in tobacco leaves (18-38 µg/kg) (Gräf & Diehl, 1966), and it has been detected in algae (Chlorella vulgaris) (Borneff et al., 1968).

3. Biological Data Relevant to the Evaluation of Carcinogenic Risk to Man

3.1 Carcinogenicity and related studies in animals

(a) Skin application

Mouse: Groups of 20 female Swiss-albino Ha/ICR/Mil mice were painted with IP either in dioxane or in acetone, thrice weekly for 12 months. Solutions of 0.05 or 0.1% dioxane produced no tumours. An identical treatment with either 0.05 or 0.1% concentration of benzo(a)pyrene in dioxane produced papillomas and carcinomas in more than 80% of the animals within seven months. A dose-response effect was detected among the groups given IP in acetone. Concentrations of 0.01 and 0.05% produced no tumours (at least half of the animals were alive at one year); a concentration of 0.1% produced a total of six papillomas and three carcinomas, the first tumours appearing at nine months. A concentration of 0.5% produced a total of seven papillomas and five carcinomas, the first tumours appearing at three months. The same experiment demonstrated that 10 paintings at two-day intervals for a total dose of 250 µg initiated skin carcinogenesis. In 30 mice subsequently treated with croton oil in acetone, a total of 10 papillomas in five animals was produced (Hoffmann & Wynder, 1966).

(b) Subcutaneous and/or intramuscular administration

Mouse: Three injections of 0.6 mg IP in olive oil at one month intervals were given to 14 XVIInc/Z mice of each sex. Ten males developed sarcomas within 265 days, whereas only one female developed a sarcoma within 145 days (Lacassagne et al., 1963).

3.2 Other relevant biological data

None were available to the Working Group.

3.3 Observations in man

None were available to the Working Group.

4. Comments on Data Reported and Evaluation

4.1 Animal data

IP is a complete carcinogen and an initiator for skin carcinogenesis in the mouse. It produces local sarcomas in the same species after subcutaneous injection. It seems to be of lower potency as a skin carcinogen than benzo(a)pyrene. It has not been tested by other routes in the mouse or in other species.

4.2 Human data

No case reports or epidemiological studies on the significance of IP exposure to man are available. However, coal-tar and other materials which are known to be carcinogenic to man may contain IP. The substance has also been detected in other environmental situations. The possible contribution of polycyclic aromatic hydrocarbons from some environmental sources to the overall carcinogenic risk to man is discussed in the preamble.

5. References

Ayres, C.I. & Thornton, R.E. (1965) Determination of benzo(a)pyrene and related compounds in cigarette smoke. Beitr. Tabakforsch., 3, 285

Badger, G.M., Donnelly, J.K. & Spotswood, T.M. (1965) The formation of aromatic hydrocarbons at high temperatures. XXIV. The pyrolysis of some tobacco constituents. Aust. J. Chem., 18, 1249

Borneff, J. & Fábián, B. (1966) Kanzerogene Substanzen in Speisefett und -öl. Arch. Hyg. (Muenchen), 150, 485

Borneff, J. & Fischer, R. (1962) Kanzerogene Substanzen in Wasser und Boden. XI. Polyzyklische, aromatische Kohlenwasserstoffe in Walderde. Arch. Hyg. (Muenchen), 146, 430

Borneff, J. & Fischer, R. (1963) Kanzerogene Substanzen in Wasser und Boden. XII. Polyzyklischer aromatische Kohlenwasserstoffe in Oberflächenwasser. Arch. Hyg. (Muenchen), 146, 572

Borneff, J. & Kunte, H. (1964) Kanzerogene Substanzen in Wasser und Boden. XVI. Nachweis von polyzyklischen Aromaten in Wasserproben durch direkte Extraktion. Arch. Hyg. (Muenchen), 148, 585

Borneff, J. & Kunte, H. (1965) Kanzerogene Substanzen in Wasser und Boden. XVII. Uber die Herkunft und Bewertung der polyzyklischen aromatischen Kohlenwasserstoffe im Wasser. Arch. Hyg. (Muenchen), 149, 226

Borneff, J. & Kunte, H. (1967) Kanzerogene Substanzen in Wasser und Boden. XIX. Wirkung der Abwasserreinigung auf polyzyklische Aromaten. Arch. Hyg. (Muenchen), 151, 202

Borneff, J. & Kunte, H. (1969) Kanzerogene Substanzen in Wasser und Boden. XXVI. Routinemethode zur Bestimmung von polyzyklischen Aromaten im Wasser. Arch. Hyg. (Muenchen), 153, 220

Borneff, J., Selenka, F., Kunte, H. & Maximos, A. (1968) Studies on the formation of polycyclic aromatic hydrocarbons in plants. Environ. Res., 2, 22

Chakraborty, B.B. & Long, R. (1967) Gas chromatographic analysis of polycyclic aromatic hydrocarbons in soot samples. Environ. Sci. Techn., 1, 828

Clar, E. (1964) Polycyclic Hydrocarbons, Vol. 2, London, New York, Academic Press; Berlin, Göttingen, Heidelberg, Springer-Verlag, p. 329

Colucci, J.M. & Begeman, C.R. (1965) The automotive contribution to air-borne polynuclear aromatic hydrocarbons in Detroit. J. air Pollut. Control Ass., 15, 113

Dikun, P.P. (1967) The appearance of polycyclic aromatic hydrocarbons and of other materials in polluted air by quasi linear fluorescence spectra. Zh. Prikl. Spektrosk., 6, 202

Fábián, B. (1968a) Kanzerogene Substanzen in Speisefett und -öl. IV. Untersuchungen an Margarine, Pflanzenfett und Butter. Arch. Hyg. (Muenchen), 152, 231

Fábián, B. (1968b) Kanzerogene Substanzen in Speisefett und -öl. V. Untersuchungen an verschieden zubereiteten Bratwürsten. Arch. Hyg. (Muenchen), 152, 251

Fábián, B. (1969) Kanzerogene Substanzen in Speisefett und -öl. VI. Weitere Untersuchungen an Margarine und Schokolade. Arch. Hyg. (Muenchen), 153, 21

Fischer, R. (1970) Spektrophotometrisches Verfahren zur raschen Beurteilung von Russen auf ihren Gehalt an polycyclischen, aromatischen Kohlenwasserstoffen. Z. analyt. Chem., 249, 110

Fritz, W. (1968a) Zur Bildung cancerogener Kohlenwasserstoffe bei der thermischen Behandlung von Lebensmitteln. II. Das Rösten von Bohnenkaffee und Kaffee-Ersatzstoffen. Nahrung, 12, 799

Fritz, W. (1968b) Zur Bildung cancerogener Kohlenwasserstoffe bei der thermischen Behandlung von Lebensmitteln. IV. Der Einfluss des Frittierens. Nahrung, 12, 809

Fritz, W. (1969) Zur Lösungsverhalten der Polyaromaten beim Kochen von Kaffee-Ersatzstoffen und Bohnenkaffee. Dtsch. Lebensmitt.-Rdsch., 65, 83

Gräf, W. & Diehl, H. (1966) Über den naturbedingten Normalpegel kanzerogener polycyclischer Aromaten und seine Ursache. Arch. Hyg. (Muenchen), 150, 49

Hoffmann, D. & Wynder, E.L. (1962a) A study of air pollution carcinogenesis. II. The isolation and identification of polynuclear aromatic hydrocarbons from gasoline engine exhaust condensate. Cancer, 15, 93

Hoffmann, D. & Wynder, E.L. (1962b) Analytical and biological studies on gasoline engine exhaust. Nat. Cancer Inst. Monogr., 9, 91

Hoffmann, D. & Wynder, E.L. (1966) Beitrag zur carcinogenen Wirkung von Dibenzopyrenen. Z. Krebsforsch., 68, 137

Lacassagne, A., Buu-Hoi, N.P., Zajdela, F., Lavit-Lamy, D. & Chalvet, O. (1963) Activité cancérogène d'hydrocarbures aromatiques polycycliques à noyau fluoranthène. Un. int. Cancr. Acta, 19, 490

Lang, K.F. & Buffleb, H. (1957) Die Pyrolyse eines Gemisches von Benzol und Pyren. Chem. Ber., 90, 2894

Lang, K.F., Buffleb, H. & Schweym, E. (1959) Über die Gewinnung neuer Kohlenwasserstoffe aus den höchstsiedenden Anteilen des Steinkohlenteers. Brennstoff-Chem., 40, 369

Matsushita, H., Esumi, Y. & Yamada, K. (1970) Identification of polynuclear hydrocarbons in air pollutants. Bunseki Kagaku, 19, 951

Reckner, L.R., Scott, W.E. & Biller, W.F. (1965) The composition and odor of diesel exhaust. Proc. amer. petrol. Inst., 45, 133

Sawicki, E., Hauser, T.R. & Stanley, T.W. (1960) Ultraviolet, visible and fluorescence spectral analysis of polynuclear hydrocarbons. Int. J. air Pollut., 2, 253

Scassellati-Sforzolini, G., Pascasio, F., Mastrandrea, F. & Savino, A. (1967) Attività cancerigena del fumo di sigaretta. Quantificazione degli idrocarburi aromatici policiclici presenti nella porzione aspirata. Riv. ital. Igiene, 27, 175

Wallcave, L., Garcia, H., Feldmann, R., Lijinsky, W. & Shubik, P. (1971) Skin tumorigenesis in mice by petroleum asphalts and coal-tar pitches of known polynuclear aromatic hydrocarbon content. Toxicol. appl. Pharmacol., 18, 41

Wynder, E.L. & Hoffmann, D. (1963) Ein experimenteller Beitrag zur Tabakrauchkanzerogenese. Dtsch. med. Wschr., 88, 623

HETEROCYCLIC COMPOUNDS

BENZ(c)ACRIDINE*

1. Chemical and Physical Data

1.1 Synonyms

Chem. Abstr. No.: 225-51-4

3,4-Benzacridine; α-Chrysidine; α-Naphthacridine; B(c)AC

1.2 Chemical formula and molecular weight

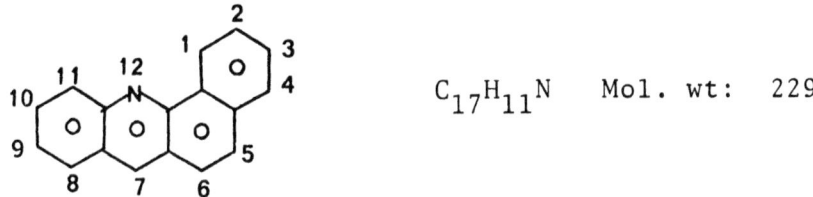

$C_{17}H_{11}N$ Mol. wt: 229

1.3 Chemical and physical properties of the pure substance

(a) Description: Yellow needles

(b) Melting-point: 108°C (needles from aqueous ethanol)

(c) Absorption spectroscopy: The ultra-violet absorption spectrum of the compound dissolved in water or ethanol appears in Perkampus et al. (1971).

(d) Solubility and/or volatility: Soluble in common organic solvents.

(e) pKa: 3.24 (Pagès-Flon et al., 1953)

(f) Chemical reactivity: Benz(c)acridine (B(c)AC) reacts in general as an acridine. For a review of the reactivity of acridines see Acheson (1956).

---

*Considered by the Working Group in Lyon, December 1972.

2. Use and Occurrence

(<u>a</u>) <u>Analytical methods</u>

Various techniques have been described for the separation, identification and quantitative determination of polynuclear aza aromatic compounds, including B(c)AC, in air, cigarette smoke and motor exhaust gases. These include paper chromatography (Luly & Sakodynski, 1965; Sawicki & Pfaff, 1965; Lederer & Roch, 1967); column chromatography (Sawicki et al., 1965d); thin-layer chromatography (Sawicki et al., 1965d; Stanley et al., 1968; Keefer & Johnson, 1970); gas chromatography (Alberini et al., 1967; Searl et al., 1970); paper and thin-layer electrophoresis (Sawicki et al., 1967); spectrofluorimetry (Sawicki et al., 1965d; Stanley et al., 1968); and spectrophotometry (Sawicki et al., 1965c; Searl et al., 1970). An improvement in the isolation of B(c)AC from tobacco smoke condensate is reported by Rothwell & Whitehead (1969). In general, the aza heterocyclics are separated chromatographically prior to determination by spectrophotometry or spectrofluorimetry.

(<u>b</u>) <u>Occurrence</u>

<u>Exhaust</u>: The level of 200 µg/1000 m^3 B(c)AC found in motor exhaust gas is low compared with those of polycyclic aromatic hydrocarbons (Sawicki et al., 1965b).

<u>Air</u>: B(c)AC has been found present at a concentration of 0-15 µg/1000 m^3 in airborne particles samples from 50 cities in the USA in 1966 (Stanley et al., 1968), whilst Sawicki et al. (1965a) report an average atmospheric level of 0.6 µg/1000 m^3 in the average urban atmosphere in the USA in 1963.

Occupational exposure: Sawicki et al. (1965d) describe the presence of B(c)AC together with 24 other aza heterocyclics and eight polycyclic aromatic hydrocarbons in various air pollution source effluents. Concentrations of 15 mg/1000 m^3 in domestic coal combustion stack effluent, 18 and 60 mg/1000 m^3 in petroleum refinery incinerator effluents and 0.12 mg/1000 m^3 in air polluted with coal-tar pitch were found (Sawicki et al., 1965c). Searl et al. (1970) were unable to detect B(c)AC in coke oven effluent, but Smith (1970) found less than 2 µg by determination of the composition of coal-tar pitch volatiles of 20 different coke plants. Kruber (1941) detected 8 g of B(c)AC in 1 kg of a coal-tar pitch fraction.

3. Biological Data Relevant to the Evaluation of Carcinogenic Risk to Man

3.1 Carcinogenicity and related studies in animals

(a) Skin application

Mouse: A solution of 0.3% B(c)AC in benzene was applied thrice weekly to the skin of 64 mice; the first skin tumours appeared at 400 days, and five epitheliomas developed in 14 mice surviving 470 days (Hakim, 1968). When 24 mice were given the same treatment combined with 0.5% croton oil in acetone once weekly, 18 survived 180 days, and two-thirds of those surviving the period of tumour induction developed epitheliomas (Hakim, 1968).

(b) Other experimental systems

Bladder implantation: Paraffin wax pellets containing B(c)AC implanted into the bladders of 58 rats induced 29 bladder papillomas, eight of which were malignant (Hakim, 1968); only two out of 64 rats given control pellets developed benign papillomas.

3.2 Other relevant biological data

None were available to the Working Group.

3.3 Observations in man

None were available to the Working Group.

4. Comments on Data Reported and Evaluation

4.1 Animal data

B(c)AC produced skin tumours in mice treated topically and bladder tumours in rats following local paraffin wax pellet implantation. It has not been tested in other species or by other routes.

4.2 Human data

No case reports or epidemiological studies on the significance of B(c)AC exposure to man are available. However, coal-tar and other materials which are known to be carcinogenic to man may contain B(c)AC. The substance has also been detected in other environmental situations. The possible contribution of heterocyclic compounds from some environmental sources to the overall carcinogenic risk to man is discussed in the preamble.

5. References

Acheson, R.M. (1956) The chemistry of heterocyclic compounds. Vol. 9. Acridines. New York, Interscience

Alberini, G., Cantuti, V. & Cartoni, G.P. (1967) Gas chromatography of heterocyclic nitrogen compounds and their evaluation in atmospheric dusts. In: Littlewood, A.B., ed., Gas Chromatography 1966. Proceedings of the Sixth International Symposium on Gas Chromatography and Associated Techniques, Rome, London, Institute of Petroleum, p. 258

Hakim, S.A.E. (1968) Sanguinarine - a carcinogenic contaminant in Indian edible oils. Indian J. Cancer, 5, 183

Keefer, L.K. & Johnson, D.E. (1970) Magnesium hydroxide as a thin-layer chromatographic adsorbent. II. A unique system for separating polynuclear aza aromatic compounds. J. Chromat., 47, 20

Kruber, O. (1941) Zur Kenntis der Chrysen-Fraktion des Steinkohlenteerpechs. Ber., 74B, 1688

Lederer, M. & Roch, G. (1967) Paper chromatography of some aza heterocyclic hydrocarbons. J. Chromat., 31, 618

Luly, A.M. & Sakodynski, K. (1965) A paper chromatographic study of aza heterocyclic hydrocarbons using aqueous solvents. J. Chromat., 19, 624

Pagès-Flon, M., Buu-Hoï, N.P. & Daudel, R. (1953) Etude d'une relation entre pK et pouvoir cancérogène pour deux séries de benzacridines. C.R. Acad. Sci. (Paris), 236, 2182

Perkampus, H.H., Sandeman, I. & Timmons, C.J., eds. (1971) DMS UV Atlas of Organic Compounds, Vol. V, Weinheim, Verlag Chemie; London, Butterworths, H8/T3

Rothwell, K. & Whitehead, J.K. (1969) A method for the concentration of basic polycyclic heterocyclic compounds and the separation of polycyclic aromatic hydrocarbons from cigarette smoke condensate. Chem. and Ind., 1628

Sawicki, E. & Pfaff, J.D. (1965) Analysis for aromatic compounds on paper and thin-layer chromatograms by spectrophotophosphorimetry. Application to air pollution. Analyt. Chim. Acta, 32, 521

Sawicki, E., McPherson, S.P., Stanley, T.W., Meeker, J. & Elbert, W.C. (1965a) Quantitative composition of the urban atmosphere in terms of polynuclear aza heterocyclic compounds and aliphatic and polynuclear aromatic hydrocarbons. Int. J. air wat. Pollut., 9, 515

Sawicki, E., Meeker, J.E. & Morgan, M. (1965b) Polynuclear aza compounds in automotive exhaust. Arch. environ. Hlth, 11, 773

Sawicki, E., Meeker, J.E. & Morgan, M. (1965c) The quantitative composition of air pollution source effluents in terms of aza heterocyclic compounds and polynuclear aromatic hydrocarbons. Int. J. air wat. Pollut., 9, 291

Sawicki, E., Stanley, T.W. & Elbert, W.C. (1965d) Characterization of polynuclear aza heterocyclic hydrocarbons separated by column and thin-layer chromatography from air pollution source particulates. J. Chromat., 18, 512

Sawicki, E., Guyer, M. & Engel, C.R. (1967) Paper and thin-layer electrophoretic separation of polynuclear aza heterocyclic compounds. J. Chromat., 30, 522

Searl, T.D., Cassidy, F.J., King, W.H. & Brown, R.A. (1970) An analytical method for polynuclear aromatic compounds in coke oven effluents by combined use of gas chromatography and ultraviolet absorption spectrometry. Analyt. Chem., 42, 954

Smith, W.M. (1970) Evaluation of coke oven emissions. Yb. amer. Iron Steel Inst., 163

Stanley, T.W., Morgan, M.J. & Grisby, E.M. (1968) Application of a rapid thin-layer chromatographic procedure to the determination of benzo(a)pyrene, benz(c)acridines, and 7H-benz(d,e)anthracen-7-one in airborne particulates from many American cities. Environ. Sci. Technol., 2, 699

DIBENZ(a,h)ACRIDINE*

1. Chemical and Physical Data

1.1 Synonyms

Chem. Abstr. No.: 226-36-8

1,2,5,6-Dibenzacridine: 1,2,5,6-Dinaphthacridine; DB(a,h)AC

1.2 Chemical formula and molecular weight

$C_{21}H_{13}N$ Mol. wt: 279

1.3 Chemical and physical properties of the pure substance

(a) Description: Yellow crystals

(b) Melting-point: 228°C

(c) Absorption spectroscopy: The ultra-violet absorption spectrum of the compound dissolved in ethanol is contained in Perkampus et al. (1968). The infra-red absorption spectrum is described in Pouchert (1970).

(d) Solubility and/or volatility: Sparingly soluble in ethanol.

(e) Chemical reactivity: Dibenz(a,h)acridine (DB(a,h)AC) reacts in general as an acridine. For the reactivity of acridines, see Acheson (1956).

---

* Considered by the Working Group in Lyon, December 1972.

2. Use and Occurrence

(a) Analytical methods

Techniques have been developed for the separation, identification and estimation of DB(a,h)AC in air, cigarette smoke and motor exhaust gases. These include paper chromatography (Van Duuren, 1962; Sawicki & Pfaff, 1965; Lederer & Roch, 1967); column chromatography (Sawicki et al., 1965d); thin-layer chromatography (Sawicki et al., 1965d; Keefer & Johnson, 1970); and spectrofluorimetry and spectrophotometry (Sawicki et al., 1965c,d). A gel chromatographic separation method is described by Klimisch & Reese (1972).

(b) Occurrence

Exhaust: Levels below 300 µg/kg of benzene soluble fraction have been found in motor exhaust gas (Sawicki et al., 1965b).

Air: DB(a,h)AC was found present at 0.08 µg/1000 m^3 of an average urban atmosphere in the USA in 1963 (Sawicki et al., 1965a).

Cigarette smoke: DB(a,h)AC occurs in cigarette smoke condensate at a concentration of 0.01 µg/100 cigarettes (Van Duuren et al., 1960). Wynder & Hoffmann (1963, 1964) failed to detect DB(a,h)AC in cigarette smoke.

Pyrolysis: Pyrolysis of pyridine and nicotine at 750°C leads to the formation of DB(a,h)AC in smaller amounts than of dibenz(a,j)acridine (Van Duuren et al., 1960). They suggested that DB(a,h)AC may be formed in the burning cigarette from pyridine, nicotine and other substituted pyridine bases.

Occupational exposure: Examination of several air pollution source effluents revealed DB(a,h)AC levels of 17 mg/1000 m^3 of gas in domestic coal combustion stack effluent, <0.12 and 0.7 mg/1000 m^3 of gas in petroleum refinery incinerator effluents and 0.01 mg/1000 m^3 in air polluted by coal-tar pitch (Sawicki et al., 1965c).

3. Biological Data Relevant to the Evaluation of Carcinogenic Risk to Man

3.1 Carcinogenicity and related studies in animals

(a) Oral administration

Mouse: Of 10 mice given 5 mg DB(a,h)AC weekly, one mouse developed an epithelioma and papilloma of the forestomach and one other mouse also showed stomach papillomas over a period of 627 days. In the same study dibenz(a,j)acridine gave negative results (Badger et al., 1940).

(b) Skin application

Mouse: Of 10 mice treated with a 0.3% solution of DB(a,h)AC in benzene twice weekly, seven survived six months, and over 349 days of observation one developed an epithelioma (Barry et al., 1935). Of 30 mice painted with a 0.3% solution in benzene twice weekly, 12 survived one year, and over 482 days of observation four developed epitheliomas and two papillomas (Barry et al., 1935). Of 10 mice painted with a saturated solution in acetone, two developed tumours over 28 weeks (Orr, 1938). Of 40 mice painted with a 0.3% solution in benzene twice weekly, five developed epitheliomas and two had papillomas over 482 days (Badger et al., 1940).

(c) Subcutaneous and/or intramuscular administration

Mouse: All of 20 A mice given a single injection of 0.5 mg DB(a,h)AC in 0.1 ml tricaprylin developed multiple lung tumours but no local sarcomas by 14 weeks after injection, while all of 14 mice given a single injection of 1 mg in 0.3 ml sesame oil developed multiple lung tumours but no local sarcomas 40 weeks after injection. Of 19 controls only four mice developed single lung tumours (Andervont & Shimkin, 1940). In a previous study, of 19 mice injected with 1 mg DB(a,h)AC in sesame oil in the groin, 13 survived 168 days and eight developed sarcomas between 168 and 240 days (Bachmann et al., 1937).

(d) Other experimental systems

Intravenous administration: Groups of 10-13 mice were given 0.25 mg DB(a,h)AC as an aqueous suspension and were killed after eight, 14 or 20 weeks. Multiple lung tumours developed in three mice out of 10, nine out of 13 and 11 out of 12 survivors at the stated periods (Andervont & Shimkin, 1940). In 20 controls, single lung tumours developed in one out of 20 after eight weeks, in three out of 20 after 14 weeks and in four out of 19 after 20 weeks.

3.2 Other relevant biological data

No data were available to the Working Group.

3.3 Observations in man

No data were available to the Working Group.

4. Comments on Data Reported and Evaluation

4.1 Animal data

In mice, painting with DB(a,h)AC induces skin tumours. Subcutaneous administration to mice induced local sarcomas and increased the incidence of lung tumours. It has not been tested adequately by other routes in the mouse and not at all in other species.

4.2 Human data

No case reports or epidemiological studies on the significance of DB(a,h)AC exposure to man are available. However, coal-tar and other materials which are known to be carcinogenic to man may contain DB(a,h)AC. The substance has also been detected in other environmental situations. The possible contributions of heterocyclic compounds from some environmental sources to the overall carcinogenic risk to man is discussed in the preamble.

5. References

Acheson, R.M. (1956) The chemistry of heterocyclic compounds. Vol. 9. Acridines. New York, Interscience

Andervont, B.H. & Shimkin, M.B. (1940) Biological testing of carcinogens. II. Pulmonary tumor induction technique. J. nat. Cancer Inst., 1, 225

Bachmann, W.E., Cook, J.W., Dansi, A., de Worms, C.G.M. Haslewood, G.A.D., Hewett, C.L. & Robinson, A.M. (1937) The production of cancer by pure hydrocarbons. IV. Proc. roy. Soc. London B, 123, 343

Badger, G.M., Cook, J.W., Hewett, C.L. Kennaway, E.L., Kennaway, N.M., Martin, R.H. & Robinson, A.M. (1940) The production of cancer by pure hydrocarbons. V. Proc. roy. Soc. London B, 129, 439

Barry, G., Cook, J.W., Haslewood, G.A.D., Hewett, C.L., Hieger, I. & Kennaway, E.L. (1935) The production of cancer by pure hydrocarbons. III. Proc. roy. Soc. London B, 117, 318

Keefer, L.K. & Johnson, D.E. (1970) Magnesium hydroxide as a thin-layer chromatographic adsorbent. II. A unique system for separating polynuclear aza aromatic compounds. J. Chromat., 47, 20

Klimisch, H.J. & Reese, D. (1972) Des Gelchromatographische Trennverhalten von Polystyrolgel fin Kohlenwasserstoffe, Amine und Phenole. Präparative Fraktionierung von Cigarettenrauchkondensat für biologische Versuche. J. Chromat., 67, 299

Lederer, M. & Roch, G. (1967) Paper chromatography of some aza heterocyclic hydrocarbons. J. Chromat., 31, 618

Orr, J.W. (1938) The changes antecedent to tumour formation during the treatment of mouse skin with carcinogenic hydrocarbons. J. Path. Bact., 46, 495

Perkampus, H.H., Sandeman, I. & Timmons, C.J., eds. (1968) DMS UV Atlas of Organic Compounds, Vol. IV, Weinheim, Verlag Chemie; London, Butterworths, H8/39

Pouchert, C.J., ed. (1970) Aldrich Library of Infrared Spectra, Milwaukee, Wisc., Aldrich Chemical Company Inc., p. 1011

Sawicki, E. & Pfaff, J.D. (1965) Analysis for aromatic compounds on paper and thin-layer chromatograms by spectrophotophosphorimetry. Application to air pollution. Analyt. Chim. Acta, 32, 521

Sawicki, E., McPherson, S.P., Stanley, T.W., Meeker, J. & Elbert, W.C. (1965a) Quantitative composition of the urban atmosphere in terms of polynuclear aza heterocyclic compounds and aliphatic and polynuclear aromatic hydrocarbons. Int. J. air wat. Pollut., 9, 515

Sawicki, E., Meeker, J.E. & Morgan, M. (1965b) Polynuclear aza compounds in automotive exhaust. Arch. environ. Hlth, 11, 773

Sawicki, E., Meeker, J.E. & Morgan, M. (1965c) The quantitative composition of air pollution source effluents in terms of aza heterocyclic compounds and polynuclear aromatic hydrocarbons. Int. J. air wat. Pollut., 9, 291

Sawicki, E., Stanley, T.W. & Elbert, W.C. (1965d) Characterization of polynuclear aza heterocyclic hydrocarbons separated by column and thin-layer chromatography from air pollution source particulates. J. Chromat., 18, 512

Van Duuren, B.L. (1962) Separation and identification of aliphatic and aromatic carcinogens from environmental sources. Nat. Cancer Inst. Monogr., 9, 135

Van Duuren, B.L., Bilbao, J.A. & Joseph, C.A. (1960) The carcinogenic nitrogen heterocyclics in cigarette-smoke condensate. J. nat. Cancer Inst., 25, 53

Wynder, E.L. & Hoffmann, D. (1963) Ein experimenteller Beitrag zur Tabakrauchkanzerogenese. Dtsch. med. Wschr., 88, 623

Wynder, E.L. & Hoffmann, D. (1964) Experimental tobacco carcinogenesis. Advanc. Cancer Res., 8, 249

DIBENZ(a,j)ACRIDINE*

1. Chemical and Physical Data

1.1 Synonyms

Chem. Abstr. No.: 224-42-0

1,2,7,8-Dibenzacridine; 3,4,6,7-Dinaphthacridine; 3,4,5,6-Dibenzacridine; DB(a,j)AC

1.2 Chemical formula and molecular weight

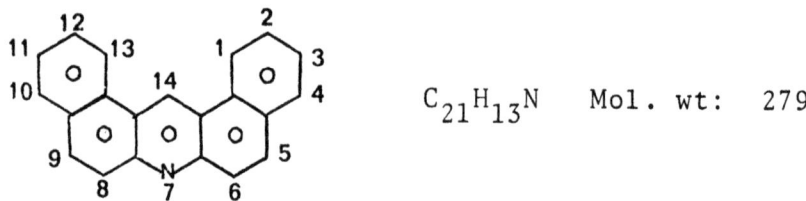

$C_{21}H_{13}N$ Mol. wt: 279

1.3 Chemical and physical properties of the pure substance

(a) Description: Yellow needles or prisms

(b) Melting-point: 216°C

(c) Absorption spectroscopy: The ultra-violet absorption spectrum in ethanol is contained in Perkampus et al. (1968). The infra-red absorption spectrum is described in Pouchert (1970).

(d) Solubility and/or volatility: Soluble in ethanol, sparingly soluble in benzene.

(e) Chemical reactivity: Dibenz(a,j)acridine (DB(a,j)AC) reacts in general as an acridine. For the reactivity of acridines, see Acheson (1956). Catalytic reduction yields Morgan's base, a molecular compound

---

*Considered by the Working Group in Lyon, December 1972.

of DB(a,j)AC and 7,14-dihydro-DB(a,j)AC (Blout & Corley, 1947).

2. Use and Occurrence

(<u>a</u>) Analytical methods

The separation, identification and estimation of DB(a,j)AC in air, cigarette smoke and motor exhaust gases have been carried out by a combination of techniques including paper chromatography (Van Duuren, 1962; Sawicki & Pfaff, 1965; Lederer & Roch, 1967); column chromatography, thin-layer chromatography, spectrofluorimetry and spectrophotometry (Sawicki et al., 1965c,d).

(<u>b</u>) Occurrence

Exhaust: A level below 300 µg/kg of benzene soluble fraction was found in motor exhaust gas (Sawicki et al., 1965b).

Air: Sawicki et al. (1965a) reported a concentration of 0.04 µg/1000 m^3 of air for the DB(a,j)AC content of the average American urban atmosphere in 1963.

Cigarette smoke: DB(a,j)AC was found to be present in cigarette smoke condensate at levels of 0.27 µg/100 cigarettes (Van Duuren et al., 1960) and 1 µg/100 cigarettes (Wynder & Hoffmann, 1963, 1964).

Pyrolysis: Van Duuren et al. (1960) demonstrated the formation of DB(a,j)AC from the pyrolysis of pyridine and nicotine at 750°C and suggested that DB(a,j)AC was synthesised in the burning cigarette from pyridine, nicotine and other substituted pyridine bases.

Occupational exposure: DB(a,j)AC occurs in domestic coal combustion stack effluent at a concentration of

2 mg/1000 m^3, in petroleum refinery incinerator effluents at concentrations of <0.15 and 1.8 mg/1000 m^3 and in air polluted by coal-tar pitch at a concentration of 0.001 mg/1000 m^3 of air (Sawicki et al., 1965c).

3. Biological Data Relevant to the Evaluation of Carcinogenic Risk to Man

3.1 Carcinogenicity and related studies in animals

(a) Oral administration

Mouse: Of 10 mice given 5 mg DB(a,j)AC weekly, no tumours were seen in 572 days (Badger et al., 1940).

(b) Skin application

Mouse: Of 40 mice painted with a 0.3% solution of DB(a,j)AC in benzene twice weekly, 34 survived six months and 21 survived one year; over 551-597 days of observation two developed papillomas and 11 developed epitheliomas (Barry et al., 1935). Of 40 mice painted with a 0.3% solution in benzene twice weekly, 11 developed epitheliomas and two developed papillomas over a period of 597 days (Badger et al., 1940). Of 10 mice painted with a 0.3% solution in acetone, one drop twice weekly, three survived 162 days; and over 245 days of observation, three developed tumours (Lacassagne et al., 1955). Two groups of 20 mice were painted with a 0.1 or 0.5% solution in acetone, thrice weekly, and after 12-14 months, 15 and 16 mice had tumours; 60% of both groups had carcinomas (Wynder & Hoffmann, 1963).

(c) Subcutaneous and/or intramuscular administration

Mouse: Of 13 strain A mice given a single injection of 1 mg DB(a,j)AC in 0.3 ml sesame oil, no sarcomas developed, but all mice developed lung tumours over 40 weeks of observation; four single lung tumours developed in 19 controls (Andervont & Shimkin, 1940). Of 10 mice given repeated injections of 5 mg in sesame oil, two developed sarcomas over 583 days of observation (Badger et al., 1940). Of 10 strain XVII mice given three injections of 0.5-1 mg in arachis oil once per month, five animals survived 139 days and no tumours appeared (Lacassagne et al., 1955). Of 20 mice injected with 0.3 ml of a 0.3% solution in sesame oil every two weeks no tumours developed over 266-310 days of observation (Bachmann et al., 1937).

3.2 Other relevant biological data

None were available to the Working Group.

3.3 Observations in man

No data were available to the Working Group.

4. Comments on Data Reported and Evaluation

4.1 Animal data

DB(a,j)AC induced skin tumours in mice following topical application and produced local sarcomas at the highest dose tested following subcutaneous administration. It increased the incidence of lung tumours after s.c. administration. Negative results were obtained by the oral route in mouse, but the test was inadequate because of the small number of animals. It has not been tested in other species.

4.2 Human data

No case reports or epidemiological studies on the significance of DB(a,j)AC exposure to man are available. However, coal-tar and other materials which are known to be carcinogenic to man may contain DB(a,j)AC. The substance has also been detected in other environmental situations. The possible contribution of heterocyclic compounds from some environmental sources to the overall carcinogenic risk to man is discussed in the preamble.

5. References

Acheson, R.M. (1956) The chemistry of heterocyclic compounds. Vol. 9. Acridines. New York, Interscience

Andervont, H.B. & Shimkin, M.B. (1940) Biologic testing of carcinogens. II. Pulmonary tumor induction technique. J. nat Cancer Inst., 1, 225

Bachmann, W.E., Cook, J.W., Dansi, A., de Worms, C.G.M., Haslewood, G.A.D., Hewett, C.L. & Robinson, A.M. (1937) The production of cancer by pure hydrocarbons. IV. Proc. roy. Soc. London B, 123, 343

Badger, G.M., Cook, J.W., Hewett, C.L., Kennaway, N.M., Martin, R.H. & Robinson, A.M. (1940) The production of cancer by pure hydrocarbons. V. Proc. roy. Soc. London B, 129, 439

Barry, G., Cook, J.W., Haslewood, A.D., Hewett, C.L., Hieger, I. & Kennaway, E.L. (1935) The production of cancer by pure hydrocarbons. III. Proc. roy. Soc. London B, 117, 318

Blout, E.R. & Corley, R.S. (1947) The reaction of β-naphthol, β-naphthylamine and formaldehyde. III. The dibenzacridine products. J. amer. chem. Soc., 69, 763

Lacassagne, A., Buu-Hoï, N.P., Zajdela, F., Royer, R. & Hubert-Habart, M. (1955) Activité cancérogène des dibenzacridines bisangulaires. Bull. Cancer, 42, 186

Lederer, M. & Roch, G. (1967) Paper chromatography of some aza heterocyclic hydrocarbons. J. Chromat., 31, 618

Perkampus, H.H., Sandeman, I. & Timmons, C.J., eds. (1968) DMS UV Atlas of Organic Compounds, Vol. IV, Weinheim, Verlag Chemie; London, Butterworths, H8/41

Pouchert, C.J., ed. (1970) Aldrich Library of Infrared Spectra, Milwaukee, Wisc., Aldrich Chemical Company Inc., p.1011

Sawicki, E. & Pfaff, J.D. (1965) Analysis for aromatic compounds on paper and thin-layer chromatograms by spectrophotophosphorimetry. Application to air pollution. Analyt. Chim. Acta, 32, 521

Sawicki, E., McPherson, S.P., Stanley, T.W., Meeker, J. & Elbert, W.C. (1965a) Quantitative composition of the urban atmosphere in terms of polynuclear aza heterocyclic compounds and aliphatic and polynuclear aromatic hydrocarbons. Int. J. air wat. Pollut., 9, 515

Sawicki, E., Meeker, J.E. & Morgan, M. (1965b) Polynuclear aza compounds in automotive exhaust. Arch. environ. Hlth, 11, 773

Sawicki, E., Meeker, J.E. & Morgan, M. (1965c) The quantitative composition of air pollution source effluents in terms of aza heterocyclic compounds and polynuclear aromatic hydrocarbons. Int. J. air wat. Pollut., 9, 291

Sawicki, E., Stanley, T.W. & Elbert, W.C. (1965d) Characterization of polynuclear aza heterocyclic hydrocarbons separated by column and thin-layer chromatography from air pollution source particulates. J. Chromat., 18, 512

Van Duuren, B.L. (1962) Separation and identification of aliphatic and aromatic carcinogens from environmental sources. Nat. Cancer Inst. Monogr., 9, 135

Van Duuren, B.L., Bilbao, J.A. & Joseph, C.A. (1960) The carcinogenic nitrogen heterocyclics in cigarette-smoke condensate. J. nat. Cancer Inst., 25, 53

Wynder, E.L. & Hoffmann, D. (1963) Ein experimenteller Beitrag zur Tabakrauchkanzerogenese. Dtsch. med. Wschr., 88, 623

Wynder, E.L. & Hoffmann, D. (1964) Experimental tobacco carcinogenesis. Advanc. Cancer Res., 8, 249

7H-DIBENZO(c,g)CARBAZOLE*

1. Chemical and Physical Data

1.1 Synonyms

Chem. Abstr. No.: 194-59-2

3,4,5,6-Dibenzcarbazole; 3,4,5,6-Dinaphthacarbazole; 7H-DB(c,g)C

1.2 Chemical formula and molecular weight

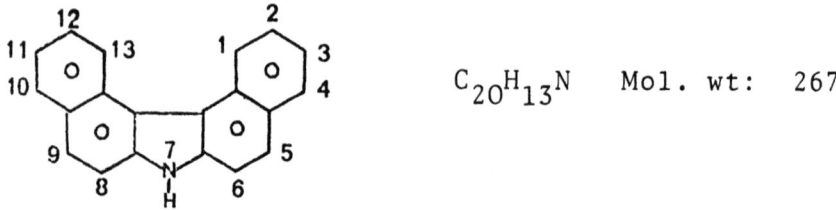

$C_{20}H_{13}N$ Mol. wt: 267

1.3 Chemical and physical properties of the pure substance

(a) Description: Needles from ethanol

(b) Melting-point: 158°C

(c) Absorption spectroscopy: The ultra-violet absorption spectrum in dioxane is contained in Perkampus et al. (1968). The infra-red absorption spectrum is described in Pouchert (1970).

(d) Solubility and/or volatility: Soluble in common organic solvents, insoluble in petroleum ether.

(e) Chemical reactivity: 7H-Dibenzo(c,g)carbazole (7H-DB(c,g)C) reacts in general as a carbazole. For a review of the reactivity of carbazoles, see Sumpter & Miller (1954).

---

* Considered by the Working Group in Lyon, December 1972.

2. Use and Occurrence

(<u>a</u>) Analytical methods

Methods for the separation and identification of 7H-DB(c,g)C in cigarette smoke condensate are reported by Van Duuren (1962). Bender et al. (1964) describe several thin-layer chromatographic systems used in the separation of carbazoles and polynuclear carbazoles and also a modification in the solvent medium leading to an improvement in the spectrometric, spectrofluorimetric and fluorescent spot test techniques. An improvement in the isolation of 7H-DB(c,g)C from tobacco smoke condensate is reported by Rothwell & Whitehead (1969).

(<u>b</u>) Occurrence

<u>Cigarette smoke</u>: 7H-DB(c,g)C was found to be present in cigarette tar in concentrations of 0.07 µg/100 cigarettes (Van Duuren et al., 1960).

3. Biological Data Relevant to the Evaluation of Carcinogenic Risk to Man

3.1 Carcinogenicity and related studies in animals

(a) Oral administration

<u>Mouse</u>: Groups of 10-30 mice (CBA or Strong A strain) received twice-weekly oral doses of 0.25-4.0 mg 7H-DB(c,g)C (total dose 7-23 mg) as a 0.125-1% solution in arachis oil. The first forestomach tumour appeared at 17 weeks, and of 55 mice surviving 17-59 weeks of treatment 64% had papillomas and 13% had squamous carcinomas of the forestomach. Benign hepatomas appeared in 19 animals (four Strong A and 15 CBA) and malignant hepatomas in a further 19 animals (18 Strong A

and one CBA). Pulmonary adenomas were seen in all Strong A mice, but in none of the CBA mice. Tumour incidences in controls are not reported (Armstrong & Bonser, 1950).

(b) Skin application

Mouse: After application of a 0.1 or 0.3% solution of 7H-CB(c,g)C in benzene twice-weekly to 60 mice, of which 34 died early, four developed skin carcinomas (the first at about 160 days) and four developed skin papillomas, over 240 days; five out of 10 survivors (182-321 days) developed hepatomas, whereas no hepatomas developed in 35 controls (Boyland & Brues, 1937). The same workers applied a 0.1% solution in benzene twice weekly to 30 mice, four of which developed carcinomas (the first at 175 days), over 321 days. Of five CBA mice painted with a 0.5% solution in benzene twice weekly, four developed squamous cell carcinomas of the skin over several months (Strong et al., 1938).

Of 24 mice painted with 0.1-0.2% solutions in acetone, 22 survived 150 days, and over 550 days of observation five showed papillomas (the first at 105 days) and 12 showed carcinomas (the first at 150 days) (Kirby & Peacock, 1946). After application of a 0.2% solution in acetone thrice weekly to 12 mice, papillomas, squamous carcinomas and one hepatoma developed after an average latent period of 110 days (Kirby, 1948).

(c) Inhalation and/or intratracheal administration

Hamster: Of 35 Syrian hamsters given 15 weekly instillations of 3 mg 7H-DB(c,g)C suspended with an equal amount of haematite dust in saline, 30 developed 42 tumours in the respiratory tract; these were mainly squamous cell carcinomas and adenocarcinomas of the bronchial and tracheal epithelium. The first tumour appeared at 15 weeks. Of 45 hamsters given 30 similar weekly instillations of 0.5 mg, 40 developed 69 respiratory tumours, predominantly squamous cell carcinomas of the trachea, bronchi and larynx, with the first tumour appearing in the trachea at 30 weeks (Sellakumar & Shubik, 1972). Comparable dosage with benzo(a)pyrene (total dose 15 mg) produced a 30% incidence of respiratory tumours (Montesano et al., 1970).

(d) Subcutaneous and/or intramuscular administration

Mouse: Three groups of 18 male CBA, 24 male CBA and 18 male A mice were given six weekly doses of 0.2 ml of a 0.1% solution of 7H-DB(c,g)C in sesame oil (total, 1.2 mg/mouse). In the first group, 14/16 animals developed local sarcomas, two out of 16 lung tumours and five out of 16 liver tumours. In the second and third groups all mice developed local sarcomas, and three animals in the second group developed liver tumours (Strong et al., 1938). Twenty mice were given 0.2 mg in sesame oil, and over 40 weeks 17 developed sarcomas and eight showed lung tumours (Andervont & Shimkin, 1940). Groups of strain A, C3H and C mice were given single 0.2 mg doses in lard, sesame oil or olive oil, and over 42 weeks of observation 17/93 C3H mice (lard), 72/133 A mice (sesame oil), 20/27 A mice (olive oil), 5/19 C3H mice (lard), 22/41 C3H mice (sesame oil) and 46/67 C3H mice (sesame oil) showed sarcomas. Hepatic changes, characterized by cyst formation and bile-duct proliferation, were also seen. Lung tumours arose only in strain A mice at an incidence of 55/78, 43/65 and 18/27 (Andervont & Edwards, 1941).

Of 20 stock mice given two single injections of 7H-DB(c,g)C (0.2 and 0.4 mg) in arachis oil, 12 survived 100 days, and over 280 days of observation 12 developed sarcomas (the first at 113 days, no metastases) and one hepatoma (Kirby & Peacock, 1935). Of 10 CBA mice given single injections of 0.3 mg in 0.25 ml tricaprylin plus 0.5 mg in 0.25 ml arachis oil, all eight mice surviving 110 days developed sarcomas, and two also developed hepatomas (Kirby, 1943). Fifteen mice were given three injections of 1 mg 7H-DB(c,g)C in arachis oil over a one month interval; seven which survived 240-382 days developed sarcomas, the first appearing at 219 days (Lacassagne et al., 1955).

Rat: Of 10 rats given 2 ml twice weekly of a 0.05% colloidal suspension of 7H-DB(c,g)C, all eight survivors showed sarcomas over 196 days (Boyland & Brues, 1937).

(e) Intraperitoneal administration

Mouse: Of 65 mice given a single intraperitoneal injection of 12.5 mg/kg bw of 7H-DB(c,g)C in olive oil, 28 survived 39 days, and one animal developed a sarcoma over 200 days of observation; liver cholangiomas were also seen (Boyland & Mawson, 1938).

(f) Other experimental systems

Intravenous injection: Groups of 10-12 mice were given single doses of 0.25 mg 7H-DB(c,g)C in aqueous suspension and were killed eight, 14 and 20 weeks later: lung tumours developed in seven out of 10, nine out of 10 and 12/12, respectively, whilst lung tumour incidence in controls was one out of 20, three out of 20 and four out of 19 at the stated periods (Andervont & Shimkin, 1940).

Bladder implantation: Following implantation of 10-20 mg paraffin wax pellets containing 1-2 mg 7H-DB(c,g)C in the bladder of mice, eight survived at least 14 weeks; three developed papillomas or adenomas (the first appeared at 14 weeks), two developed carcinomas (the first at 17 weeks) and two showed metaplasia (Bonser et al., 1952). None of the 12 control mice given pellets containing only paraffin wax and surviving 20-40 weeks developed tumours. One dog was given 5 ml of a 0.25% solution in arachis oil weekly for 12 months, and over three-and-a-half years it developed multiple papillomas (approximately 40) and one urinary cystic transitional-cell carcinoma (Bonser et al., 1954).

3.2 Other relevant biological data

None were available to the Working Group.

3.3 Observations in man

No data were available to the Working Group.

4. Comments on Data Reported and Evaluation

4.1 Animal data

7H-DB(c,g)C is carcinogenic in the mouse, rat, hamster and possibly in the dog. It has both a local and systemic carcinogenic effect. Following oral administration in the mouse, forestomach tumours and hepatomas occurred; intratracheal administration to hamsters produced tumours of the respiratory tract. In comparison with benzo(a)pyrene, 7H-DB(c,g)C appears to be a stronger respiratory tract carcinogen for the hamster.

4.2 Human data

No case reports or epidemiological studies on the significance of 7H-DB(c,g)C exposure to man are available. The substance has been detected in cigarette tar. The possible contribution of heterocyclic compounds from some environmental sources to the overall carcinogenic risk to man is discussed in the preamble.

5. References

Andervont, H.B. & Edwards, J.E. (1941) Hepatic changes and subcutaneous and pulmonary tumors induced by subcutaneous injection of 3,4,5,6-dibenzcarbazole. J. nat. Cancer Inst., 2, 139

Andervont, H.B. & Shimkin, M.B. (1940) Biologic testing of carcinogens. II. Pulmonary tumor induction technique. J. nat. Cancer Inst., 1, 225

Armstrong, E.C. & Bonser, G.M. (1950) Squamous carcinoma of the forestomach and other lesions in mice following oral administration of 3,4,5,6-dibenzcarbazole. Brit. J. Cancer, 4, 203

Bender, D.F., Sawicki, E. & Wilson, R.M. (1964) Fluorescent detection and spectrophotofluorometric characterization and estimation of carbazoles and polynuclear carbazoles separated by thin-layer chromatography. Analyt. Chem., 36, 1011

Bonser, G.M., Clayson, D.B., Jull, J.W. & Pyrah, L.N. (1952) The carcinogenic properties of 2-amino-1-naphthol hydrochloride and its parent amine 2-naphthylamine. Brit. J. Cancer, 6, 412

Bonser, G.M., Crabbe, J.G.S. & Jull, J.W. (1954) Induction of epithelial neoplasms in the urinary bladder of the dog by intravesical injection of a chemical carcinogen. J. Path. Bact., 68, 561

Boyland, E. & Brues, A.M. (1937) The carcinogenic action of dibenzcarbazoles. Proc. roy. Soc. London B, 122, 429

Boyland, E. & Mawson, E.H. (1938) Changes in the livers of mice after administration of 3,4,5,6-dibenzcarbazole. Biochem. J., 32, 1460

Kirby, A.H.M. (1948) The carcinogenic activity of N-ethyl-3,4,5,6-dibenzcarbazole. Biochem. J., 42, 1v

Kirby, A.H.M. & Peacock, P.R. (1946) The influence of methylation on carcinogenic activity. I. N-ethyl-3,4,5,6-dibenzcarbazole. Brit. J. exp. Path., 27, 179

Lacassagne, A., Buu-Hoï, N.P., Zajdela, F. & Xuong, N.D. (1955) Relations entre la structure moléculaire et l'activité cancérogène dans la série du carbazole. Bull. Ass. franç. Cancer, 42, 3

Montesano, R., Saffiotti, U. & Shubik, P. (1970) The role of topical and systemic factors in experimental respiratory carcinogenesis. In: Hanna, M.G., Nettesheim, P. & Gilbert, J.R., eds., Inhalation Carcinogenesis (US Atomic Energy Commission Symposium Series No. 18), p. 353

Perkampus, H.H., Sandeman, I. & Timmons, C.J., eds. (1968) DMS UV Atlas of Organic Compounds, Vol. IV, Weinheim, Verlag Chemie; London, Butterworths, H16/2a

Pouchert, C.J., ed. (1970) Aldrich Library of Infrared Spectra, Milwaukee, Wisc., Aldrich Chemical Company Inc., p. 927

Rothwell, K. & Whitehead, J.K. (1969) A method for the concentration of basic polycyclic heterocyclic compounds and the separation of polycyclic aromatic hydrocarbons from cigarette smoke condensate. Chem. and Ind., 1628

Sellakumar, A. & Shubik, P. (1972) Carcinogenicity of 7H-dibenzo(c,g)carbazole in the respiratory tract of hamsters. J. nat. Cancer Inst., 48, 1641

Strong, L.C., Smith, G.M. & Gardner, W.J. (1938) Induction of tumors by 3,4,5,6-dibenzcarbazole in male mice of the CBA strain, which develops spontaneous hepatoma. Yale J. Biol. Med., 10, 335

Sumpter, W.C. & Miller, F.M. (1954) The chemistry of heterocyclic compounds. Vol. 8, Heterocyclic compounds with indole and carbazole systems, New York, Interscience

Van Duuren, B.L. (1962) Separation and identification of aliphatic and aromatic carcinogens from environmental sources. Nat. Cancer Inst. Monogr., 9, 135

Van Duuren, B.L., Bilbao, J.A. & Joseph, C.A. (1960) The carcinogenic nitrogen heterocyclics in cigarette smoke condensate. J. nat. Cancer Inst., 25, 53

CUMULATIVE INDEX TO IARC MONOGRAPHS ON THE EVALUATION
OF CARCINOGENIC RISK OF CHEMICALS TO MAN

Numbers underlined indicate volume and numbers in italics indicate page.

Aflatoxin B1	$\underline{1}$, *145*
Aflatoxin B2	$\underline{1}$, *145*
Aflatoxin G1	$\underline{1}$, *145*
Aflatoxin G2	$\underline{1}$, *145*
4-Aminobiphenyl	$\underline{1}$, *74*
Arsenic	$\underline{2}$, *48*
Arsenic pentoxide	$\underline{2}$, *48*
Arsenic trioxide	$\underline{2}$, *48*
Asbestos	$\underline{2}$, *17*
Auramine	$\underline{1}$, *69*
Benz(c)acridine	$\underline{3}$, *241*
Benz(a)anthracene	$\underline{3}$, *45*
Benzidine	$\underline{1}$, *80*
Benzo(b)fluoranthene	$\underline{3}$, *69*
Benzo(j)fluoranthene	$\underline{3}$, *82*
Benzo(a)pyrene	$\underline{3}$, *91*
Benzo(e)pyrene	$\underline{3}$, *137*
Beryl	$\underline{1}$, *18*
Beryllium	$\underline{1}$, *17*
Beryllium oxide	$\underline{1}$, *17*
Beryllium sulphate	$\underline{1}$, *18*
Cadmium	$\underline{2}$, *74*
Cadmium carbonate	$\underline{2}$, *74*
Cadmium chloride	$\underline{2}$, *74*
Cadmium oxide	$\underline{2}$, *74*
Cadmium sulphate	$\underline{2}$, *74*

Cadmium sulphide	<u>2</u>,74
Calcium arsenate	<u>2</u>,48
Calcium arsenite	<u>2</u>,48
Calcium chromate	<u>2</u>,100
Carbon tetrachloride	<u>1</u>,53
Chloroform	<u>1</u>,61
Chromic oxide	<u>2</u>,100
Chromium	<u>2</u>,100
Chromium dioxide	<u>2</u>,101
Chromium trioxide	<u>2</u>,101
Chrysene	<u>3</u>,159
Cycasin	<u>1</u>,157
Dibenz(a,h)acridine	<u>3</u>,247
Dibenz(a,j)acridine	<u>3</u>,254
Dibenz(a,h)anthracene	<u>3</u>,178
7H-Dibenzo(c,g)carbazole	<u>3</u>,260
Dibenzo(h,rst)pentaphene	<u>3</u>,197
Dibenzo(a,e)pyrene	<u>3</u>,201
Dibenzo(a,h)pyrene	<u>3</u>,207
Dibenzo(a,i)pyrene	<u>3</u>,215
Dibenzo(a,l)pyrene	<u>3</u>,224
Dihydrosafrole	<u>1</u>,170
3,3'-Dimethylbenzidine	<u>1</u>,87
Haematite	<u>1</u>,29
Indeno(1,2,3-cd)pyrene	<u>3</u>,229
Iron-dextran complex	<u>2</u>,161
Iron-dextrin complex	<u>2</u>,161
Iron oxide	<u>1</u>,29
Iron-sorbitol-citric acid complex	<u>2</u>,161
Isosafrole	<u>1</u>,169
Lead acetate	<u>1</u>,40
Lead arsenate	<u>1</u>,41

Lead carbonate	_1_,41
Lead chromate	_2_,101
Lead phosphate	_1_,42
Lead subacetate	_1_,40
Methylazoxymethanol acetate	_1_,164
N-methyl-N,4-dinitrosoaniline	_1_,141
Nickel	_2_,126
Nickel acetate	_2_,126
Nickel carbonate	_2_,126
Nickel carbonyl	_2_,126
Nickelocene	_2_,126
Nickel oxide	_2_,126
Nickel subsulphide	_2_,126
Nickel sulphate	_2_,127
N-[4-(5-nitro-2-furyl)-2-thiazolyl] acetamide	_1_,181
N-nitrosodiethylamine	_1_,107
N-nitrosodimethylamine	_1_,95
Nitrosoethylurea	_1_,135
Nitrosomethylurea	_1_,125
Potassium arsenate	_2_,48
Potassium arsenite	_2_,49
Potassium dichromate	_2_,101
Saccharated iron oxide	_2_,161
Safrole	_1_,169
Sodium arsenate	_2_,49
Sodium arsenite	_2_,49
Sodium dichromate	_2_,102
Sterigmatocystin	_1_,175
Tetraethyllead	_2_,150
Tetramethyllead	_2_,150
o-Tolidine	_1_,87

www.ingramcontent.com/pod-product-compliance
Ingram Content Group UK Ltd.
Pitfield, Milton Keynes, MK11 3LW, UK
UKHW051259180426
11947UKWH00020B/1793